WRITING THE LITERATURE REVIEW

Also Available

Action Research in Education:
A Practical Guide
Sara Efrat Efron and Ruth Ravid

WRITING THE LITERATURE REVIEW

A Practical Guide

Sara Efrat Efron
Ruth Ravid

THE GUILFORD PRESS
New York   London

Copyright © 2019 The Guilford Press
A Division of Guilford Publications, Inc.
370 Seventh Avenue, Suite 1200, New York, NY 10001
www.guilford.com

Printed in the United States of America

This book is printed on acid-free paper.

Last digit is print number: 9   8   7   6   5   4   3   2

Library of Congress Cataloging-in-Publication Data

Names: Efron, Sara Efrat, author. | Ravid, Ruth, author.
Title: Writing the literature review : a practical guide / Sara Efrat Efron,
   Ruth Ravid.
Description: New York : The Guilford Press, [2019] | Includes bibliographical
   references and index.
Identifiers: LCCN 2018041861| ISBN 9781462536900 (hardcover : alk. paper) |
   ISBN 9781462536894 (paperback : alk. paper)
Subjects: LCSH: Academic writing. | Dissertations, Academic—Authorship. |
   Report writing. | Research—Methodology.
Classification: LCC LB2369 .E289 2019 | DDC 808.02—dc23
LC record available at *https://lccn.loc.gov/2018041861*

Preface

This book was born out of witnessing some of our students' frustration as they were struggling to develop a literature review. These students told us that in the past they were provided with limited guidance on the different steps involved in developing such a review. Writing a literature review is indeed a complex and challenging project, consisting of many demanding tasks. It requires the skills of identifying a topic and locating, analyzing, criticizing, and linking scholarly works into a meaningful and coherent whole. Completing this endeavor may, at times, intimidate beginning and advanced students, as well as novice researchers and grant proposal writers. We wrote this book to support literature review writers and to help them complete the process with greater ease.

We provide a step-by-step road map that clearly and concisely describes each phase of the process in order to alleviate the stress involved in writing a high-quality literature review. This road map is accompanied by easy-to-follow suggestions, strategies, techniques, and exercises that are illustrated with vignettes from our students' experiences and writing, as well as examples taken from peer-reviewed publications.

Additionally, the craft of creating a literature review does not strictly follow a technical formula. The methods (e.g., quantitative, qualitative, and mixed), structure, and style of evaluating and synthesizing prior research should reflect the researchers' perspectives, which are grounded in different approaches to knowledge and research. Considering the range of these approaches, this book focuses on three major types of review: systematic, traditional–narrative, and hermeneutic–phenomenological. It describes the features that are common to all three types, and highlights what is unique to each.

The audience for this book includes graduate and doctoral students in education, humanities, and social sciences. The book can serve as a main course textbook or in conjunction with other texts in courses that prepare students to write their theses or dissertations. In writing the book we also had in mind graduate as well as advanced undergraduate students who need to develop literature reviews for a class research project or term paper. Additionally, the book's audience may include professionals who are writing a literature review for a grant proposal, conference presentation, or for publication.

ORGANIZATION OF THE BOOK |||||||||||||||||||||||||||||||||||||||||||||||||||||||||||||||||||||||||||||||||||||||||||||||||||

For clarity and for practical reasons, the book is organized around an easy-to-follow sequence for developing the literature review. The description of the process progresses step by step through the following chapters:

1. What Is a Literature Review?
2. Different Orientations to a Literature Review
3. Choosing a Review Topic and Formulating a Research Question
4. Locating and Organizing Research Sources
5. Selecting, Analyzing, and Keeping Notes of Sources
6. Evaluating Research Articles
7. Structuring and Organizing the Literature Review
8. Developing Arguments and Supporting Claims
9. Synthesizing and Interpreting the Literature
10. The Writer Voice and the Writing Process
11. Acknowledging Sources: Citations, Quotations, and Plagiarism
12. Putting It All Together

Although we describe the writing of a review as a step-by-step task, in reality this process is not linear. Writing a literature review is dynamic, and different parts of the review are interconnected and inform each other. Instructors and their students may prefer to skip a chapter or go back and forth between the suggested steps. For example, they may choose to address the topics of writer's voice and writing style earlier in the process, although in this book these topics are discussed in Chapters 10 and 11.

PEDAGOGICAL FEATURES |||||||||||||||||||||||||||||||||||||||||||||||||||||||||||||||||||||||||||||||||||||||||||||||||||

In this book, we provide clear explanations of how to develop a literature review. These are accompanied by practical techniques and strategies aimed to increase the reader's skills and comprehension of the process. We include examples from a wide variety of academic journals, as well as vignettes drawn from our students' experiences and writing. The book includes the following pedagogical features:

▶ Checklists of suggestions and guidelines that enable literature review writers to assess the progress and quality of their own work.

▶ *To Do* activities that provide instructions for developing tools involved in the process of writing the literature review.

▶ Graphics that organize and visually illustrate the steps in the literature review process.

▶ Text boxes with examples that depict the different elements of writing a review.

▶ Summary tables that highlight the main aspects of different strategies.

▶ *Group Work* activities that invite students to further explore and apply the methods discussed in the chapter.

▶ Chapter summaries that review and highlight the main points discussed in each chapter.

▶ *What's Next?* sections at the end of each chapter that briefly review the chapter and offer advance organizers for the next.

▶ Suggestions of software for locating, organizing, and arranging sources and for note-taking.

▶ Assessment matrices at the end of the book for reviewing and refining the completed literature review.

ACKNOWLEDGMENTS

Our special thanks and appreciation go, first and foremost, to C. Deborah Laughton, our editor at The Guilford Press. Deborah's steady hand guided us throughout the process of writing the book as she provided expert advice and helpful suggestions. We could always count on her to respond quickly and thoroughly to our queries, to suggest solutions to questions that we raised, and to propose the necessary revisions to enhance the content, flow, and organization of the book. Special thanks go also to Senior Production Editor Jeannie Tang, who guided us through the production process. We also want to express our gratitude to Donna Rafanello, who read each draft of every chapter and offered editorial comments and suggestions to enhance the flow and clarity of our manuscript. Special thanks go to Steve McKinley, our graphic designer, who turned our amateur drawings into beautiful, professional graphics. We also include sincere thanks to the initially anonymous manuscript reviewers, Marsha Harman, Psychology Program, Sam

Extended Contents

CHAPTER 1

What Is a Literature Review?

Sue is a doctoral student in social sciences. She is about to complete her coursework and is thinking about her next step, the dissertation work. For the last 7 years, she has worked as a social worker in an inner-city community. Although she is not sure about her focus, she knows that she wants to explore ways to better utilize community resources. Her vision is to help individuals and families escape poverty, but she is also thinking of finding ways to strengthen the relationships among families and local organizations.

Sue is all fired up about this topic but feels overwhelmed by the many issues involved. She realizes that the topic is too wide and she needs to carve out a focus that is not too overwhelming but not too limited in scope. Her advisor praises her choice of topic but suggests that she read more about theories and research studies related to it. Sue remembers that she wrote a paper about social capital theory which asserts that shared values and social relationships, as well as investment in community sources, produce future benefits for its members. She believes this theory may apply to her future research and at the same time she feels that critical theory—and perhaps also critical race theory—is relevant as well. Her advisor suggests that to gain in-depth knowledge about theories that are relevant to her topic she should start working on her literature review. Reading the literature, the advisor noted, will help Sue narrow the topic of her dissertation research. The literature review will inform her about what is already known about the topic and identify areas where new knowledge is needed, as well as help in designing her own study.

Sue's example illustrates that carrying out a comprehensive literature review is a required step in any research project. First, a researcher cannot conduct the study

1

without gaining a deep understanding of the research topic and learning from the work of other scholars and researchers in the field (Creswell, 2018). Without being aware of what is already known, novice researchers might explore a research question that was previously investigated exhaustively, inadvertently replicate studies done before, or repeat past methodological mistakes. Moreover, writing a good literature review allows researchers to demonstrate the intellectual depth and scholarship needed for making independent decisions that are part and parcel of conducting any research project.

Like Sue, you may find yourself ready to start your term paper, thesis, dissertation, or grant proposal and wondering about what a literature review is, why it is needed, how it contributes to your study, and what steps are involved in conducting it. In this book, we answer these questions and guide you through the process of conducting the review.

In this chapter, we offer an introduction to the process that will allow you to successfully start the challenging and exciting journey of writing the literature review. We begin with a discussion highlighting the purposes and contributions of literature reviews, followed by an overview of the literature review process. Next, we suggest ways of constructing a plan of action that will enhance your ability to finish the work within your time frame. The final section in the chapter includes a short description of each chapter in the book.

WHAT IS A LITERATURE REVIEW?

A literature review is a systematic examination of the scholarly literature about one's topic. It critically analyzes, evaluates, and synthesizes research findings, theories, and practices by scholars and researchers that are related to an area of focus. In reviewing the literature, the writer should present a comprehensive, critical, and accurate understanding of the current state of knowledge; compare different research studies and theories; reveal gaps in current literature; and indicate what needs to be done to advance what is already known about the topic of choice.

A literature review may be a stand-alone or embedded in the study. A *stand-alone* review is a self-contained document that comprises an extensive review of the literature and provides a broad overview of the current knowledge about a particular topic. While a stand-alone review may serve as a basis for future research, the review itself is not followed by a research study. Examples of this kind of review may be found in term papers for graduate and postgraduate class assignments; entire theses or dissertations, especially those that are theoretically or philosophically based; and chapters in a book or review articles. In fact there are journals in different disciplines (e.g., *Annual Review of Economics, Review of*

Educational Research Annual Review of Sociology, Annual Review of Organizational Psychology, and Organizational Behavior) that are dedicated to publishing stand-alone literature review articles.

A more common kind of literature review is an *embedded* review that is an integral part of a study and serves as the context for the issue being explored. This type of review provides a direct connection between the sources and the problem to be studied and it has implications for the design of the future studies. The writer demonstrates how the proposed study expands the existing knowledge and contributes to a fuller understanding of the topic. This kind of literature review serves as a foundation for studies such as theses, dissertations, research projects, or grant proposals. In addition, an embedded literature review provides an introduction to scholarly journal articles, or policy and position papers.

Both kinds of literature review—the stand-alone and embedded—highlight the evolutionary and cumulative nature of knowledge creation. The progress of knowledge building depends on trustworthy interpretation of past research and scholarship. Schulman (1999) calls the ability to learn from those who came before us *generativity,* and argues that this ability is one of the hallmarks of scholarship. Only by gaining generativity and situating our work meaningfully within the pre-existing scholarly milieu are we able to create valuable and relevant studies and accomplish one of research's main goals—expansion of our collective knowledge (Ravitch & Riggan, 2017). Ultimately, "Good research is good because it advances our collective understanding" (Boote & Beile, 2005, p. 3).

While the process of writing either a stand-alone or embedded literature review is largely similar, our focus in this book is mainly on conducting a literature review that is an integral part of research projects, theses, dissertations, grant proposals, or policy papers.

|||||||||||||||||||||||||||||||| THE PURPOSES AND CONTRIBUTIONS OF A LITERATURE REVIEW

Before we describe the purposes of the literature review and its contributions to your research, we want to emphasize what a literature review is *not.*

▶ A literature review is not an annotated bibliography where you summarize and describe individual sources on your topic. Rather, a literature review synthesizes sources that relate to particular themes and guiding concepts. The difference between an annotated bibliography and a literature review is, according to Axelrod and Cooper (2012), similar to the difference between still pictures and a movie. A movie contains still pictures, but it connects them into a meaningful story line.

▶ A literature review is not a presentation of your own ideas, arguments, and assumptions. Rather, your claims should be based on studies conducted by researchers or theories put forth by authoritative scholars.

▶ A literature review is not a position paper. As you review the current literature, you should not cherry-pick sources that support your point of view and overlook references that represent opposing perspectives. You may share your position and provide the rationale for embracing it, but at the same time you should be open to acknowledging the value of different approaches and perspectives, compare and contrast different positions, and present the pros and cons of each.

▶ A literature review should not simply mirror the current literature in the field (Boote & Beile, 2005). Instead, it should aim to present the current knowledge through a fresh and creative perspective that contributes to new thinking and understanding of the topic being investigated.

Once we understand what a literature review is not, we can now turn to considering the many purposes of a good and rigorous review. In the following section we provide a list of potential purposes of a literature review. We do not rank these purposes hierarchically according to their importance; rather, we perceive all of them to be equally valuable. You may consider the following purposes according to the specific nature of your study and decide which ones should be addressed and the level of emphasis assigned to those you have chosen. Following Ravitch and Riggan (2017), we divided the purposes into three major categories: (1) purposes that set the context for the study, (2) purposes that inform the research design and methodology, and (3) purposes that identify areas for advancing scholarship in the field.

Purposes That Set the Context for the Study

▶ Clarify and define terms and key concepts used in the context of your study.

▶ Situate the topic within the historical background of your research area.

▶ Set up a theoretical framework for your study and contrast perspectives, ideas, and approaches.

▶ Recognize influential researchers and scholars and seminal studies that have shaped your field of study.

▶ Place the topic within a contemporary context and demonstrate knowledge of state-of-the-art developments.

▶ Discuss current debates, controversies, and questions.

▶ Identify relationships between ideas and theories and their practical implications.

Purposes That Inform the Research Design and Methodology

▶ Narrow the research problem to make it feasible and doable within your context and constraints.

▶ Refine the focus of your study or even modify the topic of your research.

▶ Identify and critique methodological assumptions and research techniques employed in previous studies.

▶ Uncover methodologies and instrumentation that may help you design your own study and develop your data collection and analysis strategies.

▶ Highlight deficiencies in previous research that may help you avoid similar flaws and errors.

▶ Prevent unintentional duplication of previously conducted studies or, alternatively, extend existing research to new methodology, settings, and participants.

▶ Confirm the "researchability" (Hart, 1998) of the research question.

▶ Ensure avoidance of insignificant or trivial research.

Purposes That Identify Areas for Advancing the Scholarship in the Field

▶ Summarize existing research in ways that allow new perspectives or interpretations to emerge.

▶ Justify the significance of your investigation by establishing the importance of the issue your research is addressing.

▶ Point out gaps in existing research and illustrate areas of concern or omissions that still need to be explored.

▶ Demonstrate how your research is linked to the studies reviewed and the existing body of knowledge.

▶ Indicate how your research revises, extends, or refines the understanding and knowledge of the topic.

As you can see, writing a literature review serves multiple purposes and may seem like a complex and challenging endeavor. Completing this work may, at times, intimidate beginners or even advanced students, as well as experienced practitioners and researchers. This book aims to alleviate the pressure involved in the process by guiding you with a step-by-step road map.

We wrote this book from a practical orientation that makes the development of a literature review accessible, efficient, and rewarding. We did this by focusing on each phase of the process and explaining it clearly, providing easy-to-follow suggestions, and illustrating the procedure of writing the review by using vignettes and examples based on literature reviews written by our students, ourselves, and other researchers.

AN OVERVIEW OF THE LITERATURE REVIEW DEVELOPMENT PROCESS ||||||||||||||||||||||

There are six major steps in developing and conducting a literature review, which are described in detail throughout the book. We realize that developing the literature review is not always a linear process. Rather, the process is continuous, dynamic, and interrelated, as different parts of the review are interconnected and inform each other. Nevertheless, for clarity and practical reasons, we developed an easy-to-follow sequential description of the process that progresses step by step from chapter to chapter. The following section highlights briefly what is involved in each of the six steps.

1. **Choosing a literature review topic.** The development of the literature review begins by selecting a topic of investigation that is meaningful for you and for your field. You will probably need to narrow down or broaden your topic by considering your purpose, your audience, and constraints such as time and access. The focus of your research should be stated as a well-defined question in order to create a researchable and manageable topic. This step is discussed in Chapter 3.

2. **Locating literature review sources.** After selecting a topic, you will locate sources that will provide knowledge and information about your topic. By identifying appropriate terms and keywords, developing search strategies, and searching records, you can search appropriate databases in your field of study. You may also benefit from tracing references in reviews, research papers, and books, or by asking colleagues or subject-matter experts for recommendations. This step also requires careful recording and organization of the identified sources and starting to create your own bibliography. This step is discussed in Chapter 4.

3. **Analyzing and evaluating literature review sources.** Once you locate sources through your searches, you will start by reading each source to determine its value for your research and whether it should be included in your review. Then you will document the themes and issues discussed in the literature that are relevant to your research question and interpret and summarize their contents. You will end by assessing the quality of the research presented in the study according to criteria for excellence that are indigenous to different research approaches. This evaluation process will allow you to become a critical reader and assess the credibility of the research sources and the extent to which the information offered is trustworthy, valid, and logical. This step is discussed in Chapters 5 and 6.

(4.) **Organizing and synthesizing the literature and building an argument.** In this phase, you will assemble the analysis of the individual sources into a well-structured, persuasive, and holistic narrative. We start with a description of strategies that will enable you to structure the literature review around themes and patterns and recognize how they relate and build upon each other. We then discuss how to construct a logical argument that presents your point of view in a persuasive way. This is followed by a description of the process of synthesizing the literature and bringing it together into a coherent whole. This step is discussed in Chapters 7, 8, and 9.

(5.) **Developing a writer voice and following writing conventions.** At this point, you will probably be aware of your voice as a writer, and we will discuss ways of developing an active and authoritative writer voice as you carry on a dialogue with the authors discussed in your review. We also offer strategies that will allow you to overcome writing blocks. Ethics require you to properly reference and acknowledge all your sources and avoid intentional and unintentional plagiarism. Additionally, you should pay attention to your writing style and language usage, as well as appropriate citation and referencing style. This step is discussed in Chapters 10 and 11.

(6) **Writing, editing, and refining the literature review.** Now you are ready write your literature review, which will demonstrate your ability to integrate theory and research and reveal a thorough understanding of current knowledge in your field and its implications for your research question. We summarize the different ways to place a literature review in a thesis or dissertation and offer different strategies that enhance the cohesiveness and flow of the writing. The completion of the literature review requires editing, revising, and refining your work, and we offer assessment matrices that will help you do that. This step is discussed in Chapter 12.

CREATING A PLAN OF ACTION

Reading through the six steps described above (which we call the CLAS-WE approach) could make you wonder how much time it will take you to complete the full process of writing a literature review. There is no exact answer to this question; it depends on the purpose of the review. Are you writing it for a class project, master's thesis, or dissertation proposal, or is it a part of a grant? The expectations are different for each type of review. The time frame may also be influenced by your professor's expectations, a grant schedule, or your professional plans. Additionally, the length of time required for completing the review depends on your own circumstances and the amount of time that you can devote to writing it.

Here is a story we tell our students when they want to know how much time it will take them to complete the first draft of the review:

> A pedestrian was walking to a small village. As he passed an old man sitting under a tree beside the road, he asked, "Old man, can you please tell me how long it will take me to reach the village?" The old man did not respond to the question. Angrily the pedestrian continued with his walk. Suddenly, he heard from behind, "It will take you about 20 minutes." Surprised, the pedestrian turned around and called out to the old man, "Why haven't you responded before? Why did you wait with the answer until I got farther away?" "Well," answered the old man patiently, "I had to see how fast you walk before I could estimate the time it will take you to reach your destination, didn't I?"

Writing the review is an individual endeavor that requires commitment, dedication, and self-discipline. Your ability to devote several hours each week, away from your many other obligations, to focus on developing your literature review will dictate your productivity and the speed of your progress.

Constructing an action plan will enhance your ability to manage your time and finish the work within the designated or desired time frame. Creating a reasonable timetable will help you to carefully navigate the process and realistically and practically schedule each step required for completing the literature review. Life's unexpected and unplanned eventualities may force you to modify your schedule; nevertheless, an overall project plan and timeline are essential for strengthening your self-discipline and the willpower required for successfully completing your work.

While there are many ways to develop a timetable, here are some suggestions that have worked for us and for our students. Start by going over the six steps for writing the literature review that we have outlined above. Be cognizant of your work style and your particular circumstances, and assess the time that will be required for completing each phase. Once you have determined the overall time needed for each step, subdivide that time according to the tasks involved in that phase. Remember to allow some leeway to accommodate and adapt to unforeseen delays that may occur when you implement the plan in practice.

Table 1.1 (p. 9) shows a section from a timeline plan that includes the major steps of writing the review, the tasks involved in each step, the time allocated for the tasks, the activities required for accomplishing the tasks, and a place for comments and reminders.

TABLE 1.1. Timeline Plan for Completing the Literature Review				
Steps	**Tasks**	**Timeline**	**Activities**	**Comments**
Step 1: Gain information on the topic	Initial exploration online; searching for information on a topic	Nov. 1–5	Use online resources such as Google and Wikipedia	Look for additional appropriate search engines
Step 2: Library search	Start narrowing down the topic; find information about the topic	Nov. 6–13	Meet with the librarian	Call and set an appointment

A LITERATURE REVIEW WRITING GROUP

We have found that one of the ways to enhance a writer's self-discipline and the perseverance required for the writing process is working in writing groups. To form a working writing group, find one or several people who, like you, are undertaking the task of writing a literature review and with whom you can talk about your progress, uncertainties, frustrations, and moments of insight. We suggest that you collaborate with your group throughout the literature review writing process, scheduling regular meetings dedicated to brainstorming ideas, sharing drafts, and supporting each other. Providing each other with honest and critical feedback is important; personal criticism should be avoided since it may inhibit creativity and original insights, and, in general, negatively affect group dynamics. The group meetings may include the following:

1. Begin each group meeting with group members reporting their progress since their last meeting.
2. Share some of the choices you have made, the inner debates you have faced, and the decisions you have reached.
3. Read each other's work and provide feedback, ask questions, and provide suggestions for improvement.
4. Together consider the next task you are taking on: What are some of the options for this task? Present your rationale for what you are inclined to choose and invite your peers to respond to your ideas.

While not all group members are required to be at the same phase in their review writing, each should share the goal of completing the process and helping the others to achieve this goal.

With our recognition of the value and contribution of working in groups, we acknowledge that for some of our students working in a group is a luxury they cannot afford due to their tight schedule. If you are one of those students, you may treat the ideas for literature review group work that are spread throughout the book as a mere recommendation.

A DESCRIPTION OF THE BOOK

The craft of creating a literature review is not solely a technical formula. The methods, structure, and style of analyzing, evaluating, and synthesizing prior research should reflect your own perspective in relation to knowledge and research. A literature review may emphasize a scientific and objective framework that is quantitative in its nature, or a subjective interpretation that is qualitative in its core. These perspectives may be grounded in different approaches to knowledge. For example, writers who promote the quantitative approach will adopt a scientific and technical framework and aim to demonstrate an objective and unbiased style of synthesizing studies. On the other hand, writers who lean toward a qualitative approach may perceive the reviewing process as a conversation with the theories and research they review and emphasize their own interpretive role. Based on the writer's perspective, there are different types of literature reviews, ranging from systematic to traditional–narrative, to hermeneutic–phenomenological.

As we describe the process of writing the literature review, we emphasize how the different approaches to knowledge and research are reflected in some of the writing phases and the procedures and strategies that distinguish each. At the same time, the processes of developing quantitative and qualitative reviews have many common features and similarities, and most of the skills, methods, and strategies discussed in the book are useful in developing both. In this book, therefore, we highlight the common procedures and methods while pointing out the distinctive terminology, ways of reasoning, and style of writing that are unique to different types of literature reviews.

Following is a brief summary of each of the book's chapters:

Chapter 1. What Is a Literature Review?

In the first chapter of the book, we explain what a literature review is, why one needs to review the literature, and what the purposes of the review are. We differentiate between stand-alone reviews and reviews that are part of the study. Then we provide an overview of the literature review process. Next, we suggest ways of constructing a plan of action that will enhance writers' ability to finish their work within their time frame. This process may include forming a literature review group comprised of classmates or colleagues. The final section of Chapter 1 briefly describes the contents of each chapter in the book.

Chapter 2. Different Orientations to a Literature Review

In this chapter we explore the three major approaches to research and their conceptual assumptions. These approaches are quantitative, qualitative, and mixed methods. We then examine three orientations to writing the literature review: systematic, traditional–narrative, and hermeneutic–phenomenological. We end with a taxonomy of the literature review that will assist writers in arriving at their own style.

Chapter 3. Choosing a Review Topic and Formulating a Research Question

This chapter focuses on the first stage of the review and provides guidelines for selecting an area of interest and turning it into a topic of study. We discuss ways of choosing a topic and narrowing it down, considering the writer's audience and the significance of the topic to the field. We end by formulating and refining a research question that will guide the inquiry. We also point out the differences between formulating quantitative and qualitative questions and highlight how the different types of review— systematic, traditional–narrative, and hermeneutic–phenomenological—impact the way the questions are structured. We then describe how to write a research question and point out the characteristics of a well-written one.

Chapter 4. Locating and Organizing Research Sources

In this chapter we discuss what a literature search is and explain its purposes. We differentiate between primary, secondary, and tertiary sources and consider the kinds of references writers should look for. We outline the techniques and strategies for finding sources through traditional and digital libraries and other online databases. We end the chapter by suggesting how writers can track and record their searches and the sources they have obtained and offer ways for them to start creating their bibliography.

Chapter 5. Selecting, Analyzing, and Keeping Notes of Sources

This chapter explores the procedures involved in extraction, analysis, summarization, and interpretation of sources. Our discussion is divided into three parts. First, we focus on the process of selecting sources by scanning the chosen articles, determining the scope of the review, and using criteria for inclusion and exclusion of texts. Next, we discuss ways of identifying the sections within each source that are

relevant to the writer's topic and how to organize the chosen sections using a digital document folder. In the third part we discuss the process of note-taking where
each piece of the identified information extractions is analyzed, summarized, and
reflected upon. We also highlight options for digital note-taking strategies.

Chapter 6. Evaluating Research Articles

In this chapter we first highlight the role of a critical evaluation of the literature
on the writer's topic. We then outline criteria that may help the writer to evaluate the quality of individual study. We highlight elements of research articles that
are common to quantitative, qualitative, and mixed-methods research. Then we
focus on those criteria that are unique to the different types of research and offer
suggestions for examining the validity of each. We conclude with suggestions for
analyzing the unique ways of assessing hermeneutic–phenomenological research.

Chapter 7. Structuring and Organizing the Literature Review

In this chapter we describe four approaches for structuring and organizing the literature review: synthesis matrix, summary table, mapping, and outline. We define
and highlight what distinguishes each, examine their advantages, describe how to
construct them, and offer examples that illustrate how they might be used. Each
strategy contributes in different ways to the writer's ability to identify themes and
patterns in his or her sources, determine how they relate to each other, and discern
the similarities and differences among them.

Chapter 8. Developing Arguments and Supporting Claims

This chapter contains two parts. The first focuses on building an argument of
discovery. We focus first on constructing a simple argument that consists of three
basic elements: claim, evidence, and warrant. We then describe four patterns of
argument that differ from each other in their level of complexity: one-on-one reasoning, independent reasoning, dependent reasoning, and chain reasoning. The
second part is focused on argument of advocacy. We discuss how to conclude the
literature review by interpreting what was learned through the literature in the
context of the writer's own intended study or future actions.

Chapter 9. Synthesizing and Interpreting the Literature

In this chapter we describe the process of synthesizing and interpreting the literature. We start by highlighting the strategies that are used in traditional–narrative
review: grouping sources, comparing and contrasting sources, exploring conflicting or contradicting findings, and adopting critical dispositions. Reviewers of

all types of research commonly use these strategies. We then point out aspects that are unique to the synthesis of quantitative, qualitative, mixed-methods, and hermeneutic–phenomenological reviews.

Chapter 10. The Writer Voice and the Writing Process

This chapter focuses on the role writers may want to adopt as literature review authors and consider whether they want to use an active or passive voice. We offer different strategies for asserting presence in the narrative and describe methods for keeping their ideas separate from those of the authors they review. We then reflect on how writers may develop an authoritative voice while "dialoging" with the authors whose work they cite. We examine the preliminary writing of literature drafts, consider factors that may inhibit one's writing, and end by offering strategies to overcome writing apprehension.

Chapter 11. Acknowledging Sources: Citations, Quotations, and Plagiarism

In this chapter, we begin by discussing issues related to three leading writing styles, with a focus on APA style. We explain and compare rules for citing and quoting sources according to the chosen writing style. We highlight rules and offer suggestions to ensure that writers avoid intentional and unintentional plagiarism. We end the chapter with a brief discussion of the basic rules for creating a reference list.

Chapter 12. Putting It All Together

In Chapter 12 we review the key elements of the dissertation and thesis proposal in which the review of the literature plays a major role. We demonstrate the interconnectedness of the literature review with other parts of the writer's research. Next, we outline the different formats for organizing dissertations, theses, or grant proposals. We then provide different strategies that enhance the cohesiveness and flow of the writing. We end the chapter by offering criteria for assessing the literature review and provide assessment matrices that allow writers to evaluate their own work.

WHAT'S NEXT?

In this chapter, we defined what a literature review is, outlined its goals, and reviewed the six major steps involved in developing and conducting it. We noted the objective and scientific quantitative and subjective and interpretive qualitative approaches to the literature review and highlighted three types of review, ranging from systematic to traditional–narrative, to hermeneutic–phenomenological.

In the next chapter, we expand our discussion and describe each of these approaches as well as literature review types and consider the assumptions that undergird them. As you design your own work, understanding these different types of literature review and their methodological stances will help you make decisions that best fit your own perspective.

CHAPTER SUMMARY

1. A literature review is a critical, systematic examination of the scholarly literature written by scholars and researchers about one's own topic.

2. In reviewing the literature, the writer should (a) display an understanding of the current state of knowledge, (b) compare different research studies and theories, (c) reveal gaps in the current literature, and (d) indicate what needs to be explored further.

3. A literature review may be a stand-alone document or embedded in the proposed study. Both types are comprehensive and highlight the evolutionary and cumulative nature of knowledge creation.

4. Knowledge building depends on *generativity*—that is, situating research and building upon preexisting scholarly work and the literature review writers build on that knowledge and highlight it from their own perspectives.

5. A literature review is not (a) a presentation of one's own arguments and assumptions, (b) a position paper, (c) an annotated bibliography, or (d) a mirror of current literature in the field.

6. The purposes of the literature review are divided into three major categories: (a) setting the context for the study, (b) informing the research design and methodology, and (c) identifying areas for advancing the scholarship of the field.

7. There are six major steps (CLAS-WE) in developing and conducting a literature review: (a) choosing a literature review topic, (b) locating literature review sources, (c) analyzing and evaluating the literature review sources, (d) synthesizing the literature, (e) writing the literature review, and (f) editing and refining the literature review.

8. Writing a literature review does not follow a technical formula; rather, it reflects the writer's perspective in relation to existing knowledge and research.

9. A literature review may emphasize a scientific and objective framework that is quantitative in nature or a subjective interpretation that is qualitative at its core.

10. Based on the writer's perspective, there are different types of literature reviews, ranging from systematic to traditional–narrative, to hermeneutic–phenomenological.

CHAPTER 2

Different Orientations to a Literature Review

I t is often assumed that there is only one way of conducting a literature review, and the instructions for completing the process are frequently presented as a mechanistic endeavor. However, a literature review is a form of research (Jesson, Matheson, & Lacey, 2011). Therefore, like any research, it is influenced by the researchers' perspectives and their beliefs and assumptions about knowledge and how it is acquired (Lukenchuk, 2013; Maxwell, 2013). Writing a literature review, asserts Hart (1998), means selecting documents "which contain information, ideas, data, and evidence written from a particular standpoint to fulfill certain aims or express certain views on the nature of the topic" (p. 13). Moreover, like any research analysis, the way these selected documents are analyzed does "not emerge out of thin air. [It] is informed by, and extends out of particular sensibilities" (Holstein & Gubium, 2012, p. 5). You need to be cognizant of your own "particular sensibilities" and their implicit and explicit influence on your perception of research and on the way you review the research of others in your field.

As you start planning your literature review, consider the different approaches to research and the methodologies that would fit your review purpose best. Becoming aware of the different perspectives for reviewing the literature, the assumptions that undergird them, and the methodological stances that they present, will assist you in making conscious decisions as you design your own work and consider different choices along the way.

In this chapter, we explore the three major approaches to research and their conceptual assumptions. These approaches are quantitative, qualitative, and mixed methods. We then examine the continuum of orientations to the literature review, which range from a systematic review to traditional–narrative review and hermeneutic–phenomenological review. We end with Cooper's (1988) taxonomy of literature reviews. which will assist you in conceptualizing your own style.

One of the main purposes for conducting a literature review is to engage in the creation of knowledge (Lukenchuk, 2013). This engagement requires that the writer of the literature review has mastered two kinds of knowledge: (1) a comprehensive knowledge of what is currently known about the subject area and (2) knowledge of skills and techniques involved in effectively finding, critically analyzing, and thoughtfully synthesizing information on the research topic.

But what do we mean by *knowledge*? What constitutes knowledge and what is the best way to obtain it? There are competing philosophical assumptions about the nature of knowledge in the social and human sciences and different understandings of how it is acquired (Maxwell, 2013). These assumptions are reflected in the different alternative approaches to research that are frequently identified as quantitative, qualitative, and mixed-methods research.

In the following section we briefly describe each of these three research orientations. We highlight the conceptualization of knowledge held by those who follow each approach, their understanding of the reality of the social world, their perceptions of the purpose of research, their role as researchers, and the research process (Gall, Gall, & Borg, 2006).

RESEARCH ORIENTATIONS: QUANTITATIVE, QUALITATIVE, AND MIXED METHODS ||||||||||||||||||||||||||||||||||||||||||||||||||||||||||||||||||||||||||||||||||||||||||||||||||||||||

Quantitative Research

Quantitative researchers apply perspectives and methodologies commonly used to study natural science in their pursuit of knowledge in the social and human sciences. Following the natural science model, quantitative researchers believe that knowledge can be acquired through unbiased inquiry. The knowledge gained is cumulative, objective, and universal. It is based on observable evidence that is measurable, testable, and value-free.

From the point of view of these researchers, there is an independent social world that is relatively consistent across time and settings. From this perspective, the social reality consists of objectively defined facts that can be discovered and systematically verified.

The purpose of scientific inquiry, according to quantitative researchers, is to seek generalities and rules in the social arena, identify causes that bring about changes, and explain the outcomes of these changes. Being able to predict future outcomes based on the study's findings is another key component of quantitative research. To minimize bias in a quantitative study, the researcher must assume a neutral and objective stance and use rigorous standards of validity and reliability.

Knowledge about the rules that govern individuals' behaviors and shape society can be gained through scientific methods that include experiments, measurements, and quantitative statistical procedures. When reporting findings, the researcher provides a detailed description of the research procedures to let other researchers replicate the study in different settings using similar interventions in order to gain standardized solutions (Wieman, 2007, 2014).

(For additional explanation about quantitative research, please refer to Black, 1999; Creswell, 2018; Gall, Gall, & Borg, 2006; Gay, Mills, & Airasian, 2011; Slavin, 2007; Yu, 2006.)

Qualitative Research

The essential difference between quantitative and qualitative research is their contrasting definition of "knowledge." For qualitative researchers, knowledge is socially constructed by the subjective meanings that people assign to their reality. From this perspective, the social reality is experienced differently by individuals and communities depending on their social, cultural, and historical backgrounds. Knowledge is, therefore, multiple, subjective, situational, value-laden, and tentative. The purpose of research is not to explain the social world but rather to understand it from the perspective of the participants. Rich descriptions of the social environment through the eyes of the people in the setting allow a deeper understanding of the complexities involved.

To achieve a holistic understanding of the setting, qualitative researchers, in contrast to the "detached" quantitative observer, become immersed in the setting being studied. Recognizing that everything researchers observe is filtered through their own subjective interpretations, they approach their inquiry with an awareness of their personal history, values, and beliefs, and consider how these influence their study.

The research is done mostly through observations, in-depth interviews, and document analysis. The findings are presented in rich and detailed narrative highlighting patterns and categories that emerge through text and image analysis.

(For additional information about qualitative research, please refer to Berg & Lune, 2011; Bogdan & Biklen, 2006; Creswell, 2018; Denzin & Lincoln, 2011; Lichtman, 2013; Marshall & Rossman, 2015; Maxwell, 2013; Merriam & Tisdell, 2016.)

Mixed-Methods Research

The third approach to research—mixed methods—is based on yet another alternative knowledge claim. This approach recognizes the different beliefs and assumptions of quantitative as well as qualitative research and respects and accepts the values of both perspectives. Rather than being committed to any one philosophical conception of knowledge, from the point of view of the mixed-methods researcher, the emphasis is placed on the practical stance of what works best in conducting the study and answering the research question at hand.

Mixed-methods researchers, therefore, are open to a pluralistic approach and have the freedom of selecting the procedures and techniques of research from among multiple methods. They may assign more weight to quantitative or qualitative methods within a particular study to reflect the focus of their research question. They may assume an objective or subjective stance or both depending on the question they are investigating. Similarly, their findings may be represented in narrative and numerical formats and highlight different aspects of the issue being investigated in ways that complement each other.

(For additional explanation about mixed methods research, please refer to Creswell, 2018; Creswell & Plano Clark, 2011; Hesse-Biber, 2010; Johnson & Christensen, 2010; Tashakkori & Teddlie, 2010.)

Table 2.1 (p. 19) compares quantitative, qualitative, and mixed-methods approaches to research according to the following categories: conception of knowledge, the nature of reality, research purpose, researcher role, and research process.

APPROACHES TO A LITERATURE REVIEW: SYSTEMATIC, TRADITIONAL–NARRATIVE, AND HERMENEUTIC–PHENOMENOLOGICAL

Although there are different ways to approach the writing of the literature review (Booth, Sutton, & Papaioannou, 2016), we focus on the way literature is reviewed as a reflection of the three approaches to research discussed above: quantitative, qualitative, and mixed methods. In this book, therefore, we present the types of literature reviews on a continuum from a scientific–quantitative framework, represented in systematic reviews, on one end to an interpretive–qualitative framework, exemplified in a hermeneutic–phenomenological review, on the other end of the continuum. Between these two opposing types of literature reviews stands the traditional–narrative review that integrates different research approaches.

In the following section, we provide a short description of each of these types of review: systematic, traditional–narrative, and hermeneutic–phenomenological. We describe each in terms of its purpose, the perspective of the reviewer, the style of searching the literature, and the process of analyzing the review.

Systematic Review

Systematic review is a scientific approach to reviewing the literature that is highly structured and protocol-driven. Proponents of this style of review claim that it is unbiased, systematic, rigorous, and replicable. The purpose of the systematic review is to answer a well-focused and specific question that is formulated prior

TABLE 2.1. Comparison of Quantitative, Qualitative, and Mixed-Methods Approaches to Research		
	Quantitative research	**Qualitative research**	**Mixed-methods research**
Conception of knowledge	▪ Objective, universal, and independent of the observer ▪ Achieved through unbiased inquiry ▪ Based on observable evidence and measurable, testable, and value-free facts	▪ Interpreted through subjective meanings assigned to experiences ▪ Multiple, subjective, situational, tentative, and value-laden	▪ Is not involved in philosophical debates and does not emphasize the significance of how knowledge is conceived ▪ The focus is pragmatic and practical
The nature of reality	▪ Independent of the observer ▪ Relatively consistent across time and settings ▪ Can be discovered and systematically verified	▪ The social reality is experienced differently by individuals and communities depending on their social, cultural, and historical backgrounds	▪ Different beliefs and assumptions about reality are recognized and opposing perceptions are accepted on equal ground ▪ The emphasis is on practicality rather than a commitment to any philosophical conception of reality.
Research purpose	▪ Gaining knowledge about the rules that govern individual behavior and shape society ▪ Seeking generalities and rules in the social arena ▪ Identifying causes that bring about changes and explaining the outcomes of these changes ▪ Finding uniform and credible interventions and standardized solutions	▪ Understanding how individuals and groups perceive their diverse realities ▪ Understanding particular individuals and settings holistically ▪ Becoming aware of complexities involved in particular behaviors and situations ▪ Allowing solutions for problems and ideas for change to emerge from the perspectives of those involved	▪ Recognizing that a study may have multiple objectives ▪ Understanding that answering the research question is the central purpose of a study ▪ Valuing and embracing both quantitative and qualitative approaches to research ▪ Solutions for the problems and ideas for change are based on their contributions
Researcher's role	▪ Avoids bias by maintaining a detached and objective stance	▪ Immersing oneself in the settings being studied and being reflexive about subjectivity	▪ Assumes an objective or subjective stance or both depending on the purpose of the inquiry
Research process	▪ Following strict procedures that can be replicated ▪ Using scientific methods of experiment, measurement, and statistical analysis ▪ Presenting the study's statistical findings in numerical formats	▪ Creating rich, detailed descriptions of social environments and individuals' behaviors gained from participant observations, in-depth interviews, and document analysis ▪ Identifying patterns and categories through text and image analysis. ▪ Presenting the findings in rich and "thick" narrative	▪ Maintaining openness to pluralistic approach to research and embracing both quantitative and qualitative methods. Assigning more weight, as needed, to either approach to reflect the focus of their question. ▪ Selecting appropriate data analysis procedures for their particular research questions ▪ Presenting findings in both narrative and numerical formats

to undertaking the library search (Petticrew & Roberts, 2006). The focus of the question is often on testing theories and hypotheses about causalities and outcomes. The researcher conducts a rigorous and comprehensive search in order to identify all possible and relevant studies on the topic under investigation. The search is based on a strict and explicit protocol appraising and synthesizing empirical evidence reported in individual studies (Jesson et al., 2011). The writer of the systematic review is required to be neutral and objective in order to minimize biases and errors. Predetermined exclusion and inclusion criteria are formulated to ensure that the information gained from the sources is accurate and impartial and that well-defined methods are used to evaluate the findings of each study. In their writing, systematic review researchers appraise and synthesize empirical evidence reported in individual studies in order to reach conclusive answers to the research question. Although a systematic review may include some qualitative research, most reviews of this type are quantitative and use statistical data (Gough, Oliver, & Thomas, 2012; Higgins & Green, 2008).

The systematic review has been developed in the medicine and health care disciplines for the purpose of conducting biomedical research. Since then, it has spread to other disciplinary fields that emphasize evidence-based decision making, such as policy and education (Battany-Saltikov, 2012).

To illustrate this type of review, Box 2.1 is an excerpt from a systematic review study on primary prevention strategies for sexual violence perpetration (DeGue et al., 2014).

BOX 2.1. An Example of a Systematic Literature Review

Studies were eligible for inclusion if they examined the effectiveness of primary prevention strategies for sexual violence perpetration and were published in print or online between January 1985 . . . and May 2012. Journal articles, book chapters, and reports from government agencies or other institutions were included. Efforts were made to gather unpublished manuscripts, conference presentations, theses, and dissertations (see above). Because the focus of this review is to summarize the evidence base for the primary prevention of sexual violence perpetration, this review did not include studies that exclusively examined secondary and tertiary prevention approaches (e.g., treatment or recidivism prevention), strategies targeting victimization prevention (i.e., risk reduction), or etiological research. In order to avoid double-counting studies, existing reviews and meta-analyses of interventions for sexual violence prevention were excluded.

Source: DeGue et al. (2014).

Traditional–Narrative Review

Between the systematic review and the hermeneutic–phenomenological review stands the traditional narrative review. This style of review remains the most common method among students and researchers in social sciences and education (Jesson et al., 2011) and is at the center of this book. Traditional narrative review draws from a variety of academic disciplines and includes diverse research methods, qualitative, quantitative, and theoretical studies. This type of review surveys the state of knowledge in a specific subject area and offers a comprehensive background for understanding that particular topic. It critically summarizes theories, examines studies, and investigates methods used in existing research. The reviewer gathers a broad spectrum of the literature written about the topic and synthesizes it into a coherent interpretation that highlights the main issues, trends, complexities, and controversies that are at the center of it (Jesson et al., 2011). The author may also identify a potential direction for future research, problems that need to be explored, or possible applications for practice.

The traditional narrative review typically starts with a statement of the problem or declares the question around which the discussion evolves; this question is often broad and may evolve or reformulate more precisely during the review process. At times, the researcher may not end the review with specific answers, but rather offer a coherent understanding of how the topic is conceptualized within the current literature. This understanding may lead to the identification of a more specific research question for the study to be undertaken.

The search of sources for the review may be extensive, although there is no attempt to locate all of the relevant literature. In this type of review, the criteria for the search methods and selection and the strategies for data analysis are usually not offered. This has brought criticism from proponents of the more systematic and scientific approaches. Those critics claim that the traditional narrative reviewers may be subjective and their arguments biased (Jesson et al., 2011; Whittemore & Knafl, 2005).

On the other hand, the distinctive pluralistic nature of traditional narrative reviews may be their source of strength. This pluralistic style of review allows for a combination of theoretical and empirical studies, draws from a variety of academic disciplines, and includes diverse research approaches. The result is a cohesive and fuller understanding of the current state of knowledge on the topic at hand.

To represent this type of review, Box 2.2 (p. 22) is an example of traditional narrative review on the topic of mentoring in education and academic organizations, written by Alexandra, one of our doctoral students.

BOX 2.2. An Example of a Traditional–Narrative Literature Review

Educational and academic organizations have become increasingly interested in developing their teaching faculty, and mentoring has become one of the major tools in achieving this goal. This has led to a surge in mentoring research and an increase in the number of formal mentoring programs implemented in these organizations (Wanberg, Welsh, & Hezlett, 2003). Efron, Winter, and Bressman (2013) highlight the importance of four elements in building successful relationships between mentors and mentees: collaboration, dialogue, sensitive feedback, and a sense of trust and acceptance.

Chapter two of the dissertation, the literature review, provides a survey of qualitative and quantitative research, as well as theoretical work on mentoring. In the review, I trace the evolution of mentoring programs in the United States in K–12 and postsecondary education; examine approaches to mentoring in research; explore the nature of relationships between the mentors and the mentees; and consider the impact of culture, race, and gender on mentoring relationships. The review draws upon research from a diverse body of disciplines, including interpersonal relationships, adult education, adult professional development, educational administration, and organizational studies.

Hermeneutic–Phenomenological Review

Hermeneutic–phenomenological review draws from hermeneutic and phenomenological philosophies as a theory for exploring the meaning of text and as a method for interpreting scholarly text (Boell & Cecez-Kecmanovic, 2010, 2014). The literature is not perceived as a presentation of authoritative truth but rather as providing an opportunity for a "conversational partnership" (Van Manen, 1990, p. 76). This conversation is among scholars and thinkers, and the writer of the review is a participant who is engaged in the dialogue, asking questions and pointing out problematic assumptions. According to Smythe and Spence (2012), the purpose of the literature review is to provoke thinking among the writers and the readers. It aims at "viewing afresh" the text (p. 14) and finding in it new meanings. The writers of a hermeneutic–phenomenological literature review are aware that their engagement with the text lacks objectivity (or a neutral stance) and acknowledge that they project their own personal experiences and social and cultural background onto their interpretation of the text.

The sources for the literature review are mostly theoretical and philosophical texts and qualitative studies, as well as works of art, poetry, and other forms of media. The hermeneutic–phenomenological literature search is not a linear process but recursive and circular. The researcher starts the review cycle by proposing a broad question or focus. This is followed by the identification of relevant literature and immersion in these sources. Being exposed to the literature leads to finding new meanings in the topic and refining the original question. Thus, the ongoing conversation with the text is extended and broadened as more sources become part of the dialogue (Boell & Cecez-Kecmanovic, 2010, 2014). The search process, therefore, goes hand in hand with the reading of the literature, and it continues until the writer feels that a saturation point is achieved. This review process is defined by hermeneutic–phenomenological researchers as the *hermeneutic circle*, which creates a fusion of understanding between each individual source and the whole, between and among the different authors, and between the readers and the text being read (Gadamer, 1982).

To demonstrate this type of review, Box 2.3 shows an example of a hermeneutic–phenomenological literature review on the seminal work of Hannah Arendt, a major 20th-century social scientist (Efron, 2015).

BOX 2.3. An Example of a Hermeneutic–Phenomenological Literature Review

In my reflections on Hannah Arendt's work, I followed the tradition of hermeneutics inquiry assertion that understanding is gained through inter-subjective interactions, where the writer's interpretations are part of a larger conversation where different voices "are acting and speaking directly to one another" (Arendt, 1998/1958, p. 183). Through the dialogical character of Gadamer's (1982) hermeneutics approach, I interpret Arendt's work in the context of her contemporary European thinkers, as well as current philosophers, theorists, and curricular writers, thus creating a Hermeneutic Circle. In the Hermeneutic Circle, according to Gadamer, "fusion of horizons" is created as points of view of thinkers from different backgrounds enter into conversations with each other and with the writer.

Recognizing the limitation of theory in relation to educational practice, the orientation of the paper is practical hermeneutics in the sense that my interpretation of Arendt's writing reflects on and responds to current experience in the field of education. Hermeneutics "can lead not only to understanding but also to personal growth and social progress" (Slattery, 2006, p. 129). My goal in writing the review follows Bontekoe's (1996, as cited in von Zweck, Paterson, & Pentland, 2008, p. 119) suggestion that hermeneutic interpretation of the literature "forms the basis for grasping that which still remains to be understood." The literature review allows the reader to engage in the Hermeneutic Circle and examine Arendt's perspective on agency, plurality, thinking and thoughtlessness, judging and moral public-space in the context of the current accountability and standardization environment in education.

Source: Efron (2015).

Comparing Systematic, Traditional–Narrative, and Hermeneutic–Phenomenological Reviews

Table 2.2 (p. 25) presents a comparison of the three types of review according to the following categories: general description, purpose, review's questions, writer's role, preferred sources, and search and selection methods.

There are other types of literature reviews used by researchers. These include meta-analysis, rapid review, scoping review, state-of-the-art review, critical interpretation synthesis, and meta-synthesis. A short description of these types of review with an example for each can be found in Appendix 2A.

COOPER'S TAXONOMY OF LITERATURE REVIEWS ||||||||||||||||||||||||||||||||||||||||||||||||||||||||||||

Are you a bit confused by the different approaches to literature reviews and their different options, purposes, and techniques? Our suggestion is that you consider each of these options and then find your own path. Focus on your particular purposes in writing the literature review and the goals you aim to achieve. As you contemplate the kind of literature review you would like write and begin planning your work, you may find Cooper's (1988) classical *Taxonomy of Literature Reviews* helpful in planning your work.

According to Cooper, there are six characteristics that distinguish different kinds of reviews: (1) the *focus* of the review, (2) the *goals* of the review, (3) the *perspective* of the writer, (4) the envisioned *coverage* of the review, (5) the review's *organization,* and (6) the intended *audience*. The characteristics are further divided into categories. We briefly describe each of these characteristics and their categories, and conclude with a series of questions you may ask yourself as you plan your literature review. We draw our description from Cooper (1988) as well as from Randolph (2009), who further expanded the explanations.

Focus

According to Cooper (1988), the focus of most research studies conducted in social sciences, policy, and education centers on one or more of these four categories:

1. *Research outcomes* center on the findings of studies and the conclusions drawn from them. These conclusions allow the writer to establish the need for further research on the topic. For example, Ali, a student from Nigeria, studies literature about the topic of water shortage and implications for health, agriculture, and economy, as well as aggression among nations over water accessibility. Based on his review, he is proposing to conduct research on projects in other countries that were able to overcome similar situations.

TABLE 2.2. Comparison of Systematic, Traditional–Narrative, and Hermeneutic–Phenomenological Reviews			
	Systematic review	**Traditional narrative review**	**Hermeneutic–phenomenological review**
General description	▪ Scientific, highly structured, and protocol driven ▪ Claims to be unbiased, rigorous, and replicable	▪ Draws from a variety of academic disciplines ▪ Includes diverse research methods	▪ Explores creatively the meaning of text ▪ Perceives the review as a conversation among thinkers and researchers, as well as the review writer
Purpose	▪ Aims to answer a well-focused and specific question that is formulated prior to undertaking the library search ▪ Tests a hypothesis through appraisal and synthesis of empirical evidence in individual studies	▪ Offers a comprehensive background of a topic ▪ Critically summarizes theories, studies, and methods used in existing research ▪ Provides a rationale for the research to be undertaken	▪ Provokes the writer's and readers' thinking ▪ Aims at viewing the texts afresh and finds new meanings
Review's questions	▪ Questions formulated prior to undertaking the research ▪ The focus is on testing theories and hypotheses about causality and outcomes	▪ Questions evolve or reformulate during the review process ▪ Questions that guide the review are often broad	▪ Questions are expected to be refined or change their focus with the writer's immersion in the texts ▪ Questions are broad and often conceptual or philosophical
Writer's role	▪ Writer is neutral and objective in order to minimize bias and error	▪ Writer does not assume an objective stance ▪ At times, this approach is criticized for being biased because criteria for selection of sources are not offered	▪ Writer is aware that engagement with the text lacks objectivity ▪ Writer acknowledges that personal experiences are projected into the meanings found in the texts
Preferred sources	▪ Most sources are quantitative and use statistical data, although a limited number of qualitative research studies may also be used	▪ Includes both theoretical and empirical studies	▪ Mostly theoretical and philosophical texts and qualitative studies; also works of art, poetry, and other forms of media
Search	▪ Exhaustive and comprehensive search based on explicit and strict protocol	▪ The search may be extensive but does not attempt to locate all relevant literature ▪ Criteria for search methods are seldom offered	▪ Search for sources is not a linear process but recursive and circular
Selection	▪ Predetermined exclusion and inclusion criteria are developed to evaluate the validity and credibility of the findings reported in each study	▪ Criteria for selection of sources are not explicitly presented	▪ Criteria for the selection of sources are not presented ▪ Sources selected are those that can contribute to the "dialogue" among the authors reviewed

2. *Research methods* highlight the strategies of data collection, analysis, and interpretation involved in the different studies and the strengths and weaknesses of the chosen methodology. This kind of review writing may be used as a rationale for the writer's own research by showing that previous studies were methodologically flawed or need further expansion. For example, Jose, who is researching ways to reduce violent confrontation between police and minority groups, found that most past studies were conducted using statistical and report data. Jose believes that there are not enough studies where police officers and youth get together to discuss openly their perception of their relationship and how to improve it. Jose decided to conduct a series of focus group interviews on this sensitive topic.

3. *Research theories* highlight the existing theories that shape the writer's research topic and the relationships between them. This focus may lead to advancing a new theory or justifying the writer's choice of a particular theory to guide his or her investigation. For example, Paul, an art museum educator, is planning to study the impact of the educational programs offered at the museum on the participants. He explores how perceptions of aesthetics have changed over time from Greek philosophers to postmodern views.

4. *Research practices and applications* center on how a certain theory may apply in practice, or how a certain intervention may be carried out within a certain setting. Using the knowledge he obtained from his literature review on aesthetics, Paul designs an art appreciation program for college students and evaluates its impact on their perception of the role of the arts in their lives.

Cooper (1988) emphasizes that these areas of interest are not mutually exclusive and most reviewers will employ two or more foci with varying degrees of attention. For example, in your review you may start by describing a theory and then examine empirical studies that test this theory, and end your review by looking at the implication of the theories and the studies' conclusions for your own practice.

Goals

What are the goals of the literature review and what is the writer trying to accomplish? This is the second characteristic of literature reviews highlighted by Cooper (1988). The most common goal for writing a literature review is to present a holistic picture of the current state of knowledge on a research topic. This goal is achieved by synthesizing past and current literature and highlighting different theoretical approaches as well as relevant studies.

Another goal that may drive the writer of the literature review is to use a critical lens when analyzing and evaluating previous literature, theories, and research in a particular subject area. This goal will lead the writer to highlight flaws in the current arguments and perspectives, or in the way past research was conducted, and offer an alternative approach that will be investigated in the proposed study.

When you think about your own goal in writing the review, you may have several goals that complement each other. For example, you may synthesize the studies done in the field of your research topic and then criticize specific aspects or identify problematic issues that you intend to tackle in your own study.

Perspective

Perspective is the third characteristic, according to the taxonomy of literature reviews. This characteristic is centered on the author's approach to research, subjective orientation, and biases. As you write your literature review, contemplate the following: (1) Do you see your role as an objective and neutral presenter of the literature, or do you see yourself as a subjective participant in a scholarly conversation? and (2) Are you a critical recipient of knowledge constructed by others, or are you a creative interpreter who shares his or her personal insight on the literature? For example, when you write about feminism, are you objectively presenting the perspectives of different writers on the meaning of feminism, or are you offering your own reflections on the different theories you describe?

Your perspective may also be influenced by your inclination to adopt a quantitative, qualitative, or mixed-methods approach for your study. Each of these approaches, as discussed above, represents a unique world view about the purpose of research and the role of the researcher. While quantitative researchers tend to avoid bias by maintaining a detached and objective stance toward their topic, qualitative researchers tend to immerse themselves in their inquiry and willingly recognize their own subjectivity and bias. Mixed-methods researchers accept both objective and subjective stances depending on their particular research question.

You may want to ask yourself the following: What is your perspective on your role as a researcher and a reviewer? With which of the approaches to research described above do you identify the most? Self-knowledge and awareness of your own inclinations is essential for your literature review experience. As Maxwell (2013) thoughtfully stated, working within a research perspective that does not fit one's own point of view and beliefs is like doing physically demanding work wearing clothes that do not fit, and consequently feeling uncomfortable throughout the process.

Coverage

The next characteristic of the taxonomy is the level of coverage in the literature review and how comprehensive it should be. According to Boote and Beile (2005), the decision about what to include and what to exclude in the review process is "probably the most distinct aspect of literature reviewing" (p. 7). Cooper (1988) distinguishes between four possible approaches to coverage:

1. A writer of an *exhaustive review* intends to consider every source relevant to the topic.

2. A writer of an *exhaustive with selective citation review* sets the boundary of what references will be reviewed according to defined criteria (e.g., age group, location, or method of research).

3. A third option is a *representative review,* where the author chooses sources that are representative or typical of similar publications in a particular field. The author often presents a rationale for making his or her choice by demonstrating how the chosen work is illustrative of many others.

4. The fourth coverage option is a *central review* where the writer purposefully focuses on seminal works that are essential for understanding the topic area.

The first two categories are usually preferred by reviewers of scientific–quantitative frameworks, like systematic review or meta-analysis, and the last two are typically employed by traditional–narrative or hermeneutic–phenomenological writers. Boote and Beile (2005) recommend that whatever coverage choice you make, you should convince your readers that your rationale regarding the level of review coverage of the literature has been done carefully, thoughtfully, and purposefully.

Organization

Organization of the literature review is the fifth characteristic outlined by Cooper (1988). Writers who choose to use a *historical* format usually employ an analysis of the literature within a historical context. It provides an explanation and evaluates the implications of an idea, a policy, or a methodology within a context of the historical forces that shaped it. Such a review is typically organized chronologically. A *theoretical* format is focused on existing theories or proposes a conceptualization of a new theory regarding a particular phenomenon. Such a format offers ways of comparing the validity, consistency, and breadth of existing theories and evaluating their strengths and flaws. Another common organization is the *methodological* format, which centers on research design methods, procedures, and the results of empirical studies that have been conducted in a particular subject area.

As suggested in other characteristics of literature review described in Cooper's taxonomy (1988), you may combine different organizational formats according to your particular needs. For example, suppose your study involves the topic of ways to successfully integrate immigrants into American society. You may start by providing a historical overview of the attitudes of governmental institutions toward immigrants since the middle of the 19th century. Next, you can focus on theories that underlie different immigration policies. Finally, you can end your review by comparing the methodologies of different studies that have been conducted on this issue.

Audience

The last characteristic of the taxonomy of literature reviews asks the writer to consider his or her audience. As you begin writing your review, consider who you are writing for. If you are writing a thesis or dissertation, you may want to take into account your professor's guidelines or the expectations of your thesis or dissertation committee. If you are writing your literature review as part of a grant proposal, you should be cognizant of the criteria that will be used to evaluate your proposal. Alternatively, if the literature review is part of an article you are submitting for publication, follow the manuscript guidelines for the journals where you would like the article to be published. In addition, keep in mind the audience that will benefit from the information contained in your review. For example, are they practitioners in the field, policymakers, the general public, workplace colleagues, or members of the scholarly community?

Table 2.3 (p. 30) presents the six characteristics of literature reviews and their categories, as well as questions that may help you make your choices as you undertake the task of writing your literature review.

Although it is important to consider the characteristics of focus, goals, perspectives, coverage, organization, and audience for your literature review, do not forget to use your imagination and creative spirit when you write your review. Lukenchuk (2013) emphasizes the role and value of imagination in any research project. She describes the role of imagination in constructing one's research as the "gateway into the known and unknown, the mysterious spark that instigates our thinking and desire to pursue daring projects. Imaginative thinking frees us from the constraints of prescriptive rules and standards that dictate how to conduct a research project" (p. 85). According to Hart (1998), in a literature review the meaning of imaginative attitude in practice is as follows:

> Having a broad view of a topic, being open to ideas regardless of how or where they originated; questioning and scrutinizing ideas, methods and arguments regardless of who proposed them; playing with different ideas in order to see if links can be made, following ideas to see where they might lead. (p. 30)

WHAT'S NEXT?

In this chapter you have gained information about the different research orientations, approaches to literature review, the different characteristics of literature review, as well as an awareness of the value of imagination in writing the review.

TABLE 2.3. Cooper's Taxonomy for Choosing the Type of Literature Review

Characteristics	Categories	Questions to ask yourself
Focus of the review	■ Research outcomes ■ Research methods ■ Research theories ■ Research practices or applications	■ What is the focus of your literature review? ■ Do you have more than one focus? If yes, what are they? In what order are you planning to discuss them?
Goal of the literature review	■ Holistic picture of the current state of knowledge on the research topic ■ Critical lenses	■ What is the goal of your review? ■ How will you achieve this goal? ■ If you have several goals, how do they relate to each other?

Perspective on research and on the literature review	■ What is your role as the literature review author?	■ Do you see your role as a literature review author as a:
		  □ neutral and objective presenter?
		  □ subjective participant in a conversation?
		  □ critical evaluator?
		  □ creative interpreter?
		  □ other?
		■ Explain your choice of role.
		■ What research approach best reflects your perspective and why?
		■ Will you use a quantitative, qualitative, or mixed-methods approach?

Coverage and scope of the literature	■ Exhaustive ■ Exhaustive with selective citation ■ Representative ■ Central	■ What is your preferred level of literature coverage? ■ What are your reasons for choosing this particular approach to coverage?

Organization of the narrative	■ Historical
	■ Theoretical
	■ Methodological
		■ How do you plan to organize your review:
		  □ Historical?
		  □ Theoretical?
		  □ Methodological?
		  □ Other?

Intended audience	■ Professors or dissertation committee faculty ■ Private or public grant committees ■ Publishers ■ Practitioners in the field ■ Policymakers ■ Workplace colleagues ■ Scholarly community ■ General public	■ Who is the major audience for your literature review? ■ How will your audience affect the way you write the review?

Note. Adapted from Cooper (1988, p. 109) and Randolph (2009, p. 3).

Now you are ready to choose the topic of your review and the research question that will become your focus. These are the first steps in the exciting literature review journey. Bon voyage!

CHAPTER SUMMARY

1. Three of the most common approaches to research are quantitative, qualitative, and mixed methods.

2. *Quantitative* researchers believe that knowledge is cumulative, objective, and universal, and is based on observable evidence that is measurable, testable, and value-free. This kind of research uses scientific methods of experiment, measurement, and statistical procedures.

3. *Qualitative* researchers believe that knowledge is socially constructed by the subjective meanings that people assign to their reality. They are immersed in the study being conducted and carry out the research through observations, in-depth interviews, and document analysis; the findings are presented in a rich and detailed narrative.

4. *Mixed-methods* researchers recognize the different beliefs and assumptions of quantitative as well as qualitative research and select procedures and techniques according to the question at the center of their study.

5. Three types of literature reviews are discussed: systematic, traditional–narrative, and hermeneutic–phenomenological.

6. *Systematic review* is a scientific approach to reviewing the literature that is highly structured and protocol driven. The research question is formulated prior to undertaking the search for sources, and the researcher uses predetermined exclusion and inclusion criteria in selecting the sources.

7. *Traditional–narrative* review draws from a variety of academic disciplines and includes diverse research methods. The question at the center of the review is often broad and may evolve during the review process and in the interpretation of the sources. The writer highlights the main issues, trends, complexities, and controversies.

8. *Hermeneutic–phenomenological review* is focused on the interpretation of the meaning of texts to provoke thinking and to examine the text with fresh eyes. The writer, who acknowledges an inherent subjectivity and positionality, starts with a broad research question that evolves as new meanings are discovered while reading sources.

9. Cooper lists six characteristics that distinguish different kinds of reviews: (a) the *focus* of the review, (b) the *goals* of the review, (c) the *perspective* of the writer, (d) the envisioned *coverage* of the review, (e) the review's *organization,* and (f) the intended *audience.*

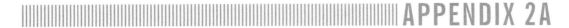

In Chapter 2, we presented three major types of literature review and placed them on a continuum ranging from scientific–systematic on one end to interpretive–qualitative on the other end, with practical–mixed in the center. In this appendix, we highlight six examples of literature reviews that represent the different points on this continuum. The scientific–systematic approach is represented by meta-analysis and rapid reviews; conceptual and integrative literature reviews represent the practical–mixed approach; and critical interpretation syntheses and meta-synthesis are examples of an interpretive–qualitative approach.

EXAMPLES OF SCIENTIFIC–SYSTEMATIC TYPES OF LITERATURE REVIEWS

Meta-Analysis

Meta-analysis is a form of systematic review that statistically combines findings from a large body of individual quantitative studies to arrive at conclusions and detect patterns of causal relationship among the variables being studied. By combining studies that look at the same questions, meta-analysis review serves as a tool for increasing sample size and thus certainty in cause-and-effect conclusions. Criteria for assessing the quality of the individual studies are strictly followed, and the findings are analyzed using standardized statistical procedures. All of these methods enhance the validity and reliability of the review's conclusions, increase precision, and reduce random errors. (For more information on meta-analysis see Card, 2011; Cooper, 2010; Cooper, Hedges, & Valentine, 2009; Makambi, 2012; Ringquist, 2013.)

Box 2A.1 (p. 33) is an excerpt from a meta-analysis study by Pallini, Baiocco, Schneider, Madigan, and Atkinson (2014) on the topic of early child–parent attachment and peer relations.

Rapid Review

Rapid review synthesizes evidence for advocating for policy, educational decision making, or time-sensitive health-practice choices. In comparison to systematic reviews, rapid review is conducted in a shorter time frame by using methods to accelerate and streamline the review process. While not using as much rigor and not attempting to find all of the sources on the topic at hand, the reviewer searches and critically appraises evidence from mostly quantitative studies and from studies that summarize a large body of research on the topic. Rapid review may also lay the groundwork for a more extensive systematic review in the future (Ganann, Ciliska, & Thomas, 2010). (For more information about rapid reviews see Ganann et al., 2010; Harker & Kleijnen, 2012.)

Box 2A.2 (p. 33) shows an example of a rapid review of the Greek Research and Development System that was prepared by RAND Europe for the Greek Ministry of Education (Grant, Ling, Potoglou, & Culley, 2011).

BOX 2A.1. An Example of a Meta-Analysis Review Study

To generate samples comparable with the 2001 meta-analysis, we used the same keywords in searching PSYCINFO, PUBMED and ProQuest Dissertations. We also scanned the references of articles retrieved and contacted researchers working in this area. Our search included studies available between 1999 and 2012. Inclusion/exclusion criteria were identical to those used in the 2001 meta-analysis: original data, measure of attachment to a parent other than self-report, collected before the child reached age 18, include a quantitative measure of children's peer relations other than self-report, feature assessment of attachment and peer relations, include data on securely and insecurely attached participants or a continuous measure of attachment, written in English or another language understood by our research team (French, Italian, Spanish). These criteria resulted in inclusion of 44 studies with 8,505 participants. Each study was coded for the following: a) attachment measure (e.g., Strange Situation, Q-sort); b) attachment figure (e.g., father, mother); c) dimension(s) of peer relations (e.g., peer-directed aggression, friendship, prosociality); d) source of information about peer relations (e.g., observation, peer report, teacher report); e) degree of familiarity (peers or friends); f) gender of child; g) mean age of participants when attachment and h) peer relations were measured; i) time between the measurement of attachment and peer relations; j) specific subject characteristics (e.g., diagnosed atypical behavior, low SES, parents divorced); k) country; l) publication date; and m) dissemination (i.e., journal article, thesis, book). Agreement on coding and application of inclusion/exclusion criteria was established by having the second author corate; agreement between first and second authors was 94%.

Source: Pallini, Baiocco, Schneider, Madigan, and Atkinson (2014).

BOX 2A.2. An Example of a Rapid Review Study

This documented briefing presents the findings of a rapid review of the Greek Research and Development (R&D) system. In considering future options for reform, and within the context of a wider strategy to enhance research and innovation in Greece, in March 2011 the Ministry of Education, Lifelong Learning, and Religious Affairs (hereafter the Ministry of Education) requested proposals for a review of the Greek research system. By necessity, the review was prepared over a short, four-month period (April–July 2011) so that it could feed into forthcoming policy decisions. For this reason we had to proceed quickly, and to ensure timely completion we focused our review on publicly funded Research Centres (RCs) under the auspices of the General Secretariat for Research and Technology.

Source: Grant, Ling, Potoglou, and Culley (2011, p. 1).

EXAMPLES OF PRACTICAL–MIXED-METHODS TYPES OF LITERATURE REVIEWS |||||||||||||||||||||||||||

Conceptual Review

Conceptual review offers a conceptual framework for the topic of study. The author of this type of review surveys the literature on the subject in order to identify and analyze the concepts involved. For example, the author may critically discuss the ways in which the topic was conceptualized in the literature, how such conceptualizations are reflected in the empirical studies that were conducted, and the implications of these conceptualizations. Often, the review writer creates a conceptual map that reflects the literature and highlights the representative authors in each area of this map. The organization of the discussion is mostly determined by these conceptual areas. The author may also organize the review around a guiding theory or around a set of competing models that conceptualize the topic. (For further information about conceptual review, see Jarret & Ollendick, 2008; Rocco & Plakhotnik, 2009.)

An example of a conceptual review can be found in Box 2A.3, an article written by Tan (2014) on human capital theory.

Integrative Review

Integrative review offers a critical analysis of existing literature by carefully examining the main ideas of a topic of interest and deconstructing it into its basic elements. Integrative reviews usually address two kinds of topics: mature topics with multiple empirical and theoretical literature and new or emerging topics. In the case of the former, the review author critiques and synthesizes representative literature in a way that results in new understanding of the phenomenon. By comparison, the writer of an integrative literature review addresses a new topic by offering a preliminary conceptualization of the topic, such as new models or a new perspective on the issue.

BOX 2A.3. An Example of a Conceptual Literature Review

The aims of this article are twofold. The first aim is to provide a clear understanding of HCT (Human Capital Theory) and its roots. To achieve this, we will go back to the philosophical origin of the theory and discuss the school of thought from which HCT takes its intellectual nutrition. To understand the roles of education in HCT, it is necessary to trace back the basic assumptions of this intellectual tradition on human beings. The second aim is to provide a comprehensive and accessible road map to those who wish to have a broad understanding of the theory and its impacts. With this article it is hoped that the reader will have the opportunity to review the major criticisms and different dimensions of the theory in a single article (Tan, 2014, p. 411).

Source: Tan (2014, p. 411).

The strength of an integrative review is its distinctive and rigorous methodology. It uses detailed search strategies, draws data from diverse studies, allows for the inclusion of multiple methodological approaches, and combines data from theoretical and empirical studies. (For more information, see Cooper, 1998; Torraco, 2005; Whittemore & Knafl, 2005.) As an example of this type of review, we quote from Park's (2010) article (Box 2A.4).

EXAMPLES OF INTERPRETIVE–QUALITATIVE TYPES OF REVIEW

Meta-Synthesis Review

Meta-synthesis review interprets findings from a group of similar qualitative studies for the purpose of transforming the findings from individual studies into an explanatory theory, a model, or a new conceptualization of a phenomenon. The different sources "talk" with each other as the reviewer juxtaposes different studies and identifies patterns and theoretical connections across them. The goal is not to come up with conclusions but rather reach a tentative theoretical or conceptual level of understanding. Additionally, the emphasis is not on evaluating the quality of the findings but rather on exploring their significance to the field. Personal reflection of the literature review writers is encouraged. (For more information, see Barnett-Page & Thomas, 2009; Lockwood & Pearson, 2013; Silverman, 2015; Walsh & Downe, 2005.) As an example of a meta-synthesis we present the thesis work of Sara, one of our master's-level students (Box 2A.5, p. 36).

BOX 2A.4. An Example of an Integrative Literature Review

Drawing on current theories, the author first presents an integrated model of meaning making. This model distinguishes between the constructs of global and situational meaning and between "meaning-making efforts" and "meaning made," and it elaborates subconstructs within these constructs. Using this model, the author reviews the empirical research regarding meaning in the context of adjustment to stressful events, outlining what has been established to date and evaluating the strengths and weaknesses of current empirical work. Results suggest that theory on meaning and meaning making has developed apace, but empirical research has failed to keep up with these developments, creating a significant gap between the rich but abstract theories and empirical tests of them. Given current empirical findings, some aspects of the meaning-making model appear to be well supported but others are not, and the quality of meaning-making efforts and meanings made may be at least as important as their quantity. This article concludes with specific suggestions for future research.

Source: Park (2010, p. 257).

BOX 2A.5. An Example of a Meta-Synthesis Literature Review

I have used the meta-synthesis review in order to gain a greater understanding of the phenomenon of homelessness among the young and its impact on their mental and emotional health. This type of review uses rigorous qualitative methods to synthesize and interpret qualitative studies for the purpose of constructing greater meaning (Erwin, Brotherson, & Summers, 2011). The qualitative studies enable an exposure to nuances and textured milieu, in all its richness and thick descriptions (Silverman, 2015). The use of qualitative findings is essential for "developing valid and culturally sensitive instruments and effective participant-centered interventions" (Sandelowski & Barroso, 2007, p. 5). Through the synthesis of common themes, metaphors, and phrases (Noblit & Haren, 1988), a conceptualization of the meaning of being a homeless child has been constructed. Thus, the goal of meta-synthesis literature review "to produce a new and integrative interpretation of findings that is more substantive than those resulting from individual investigations" (Finfgeld, 2003, p. 894) has been achieved.

Critical Interpretation Synthesis Review

Critical interpretation synthesis review is rooted in the tradition of qualitative research and is oriented mostly toward generating theory. This type of review embraces all kinds of studies from theoretical conceptualization studies to empirical research that draws from qualitative, quantitative, and mixed-methods investigations. The analysis and synthesis of the reviewed studies are based on qualitative methods. The review is an iterative, repetitive process, and the review questions emerge and are reshaped throughout the process. Although the subjectivity of the reviewer is acknowledged as a given, the review's procedures are emphasized and the criticism is directed toward procedural mistakes found in primary studies that are included in the review. Writers who adopt this type of review often analyze conceptual similarities and differences identified in the literature, question the taken-for-granted assumptions on problem definition, and examine the political, social, and cultural influences on the choice of proposed solutions. (For more information, see Barnett-Page & Thomas, 2009; Booth et al., 2016; Dixon-Woods et al., 2006; Gough, 2007; Silverman, 2015.)

An example of a critical interpretation synthesis review can be found in an unpublished literature review written by Janice, a doctoral student in curriculum studies (Box 2A.6, p. 37).

BOX 2A.6. An Example of a Critical Interpretation Synthesis Review

Since the report of Joseph Mayer-Rice in 1912 (Alan, 1984), the quality of students' learning experience in school and their academic success has been connected to the quality of their teachers. Today, in the environment of accountability and standardization policies, this connection is narrowed to measure teachers' input and test students output. As a principal of a high poverty urban elementary school for 14 years, I've never wavered in my belief that teachers are the most critical factor in accelerating student achievement. I have experienced the effects of the waves of school reform aimed to improve our educational system and have seen the impact on teachers' professional identity, emotional experience, and commitment.

A critical interpretation synthesis review approach was utilized to critically appraise and synthesize the literature on educational reforms and their impact on changing teachers' practice, beliefs about teaching, and professional identity. In this study, I will briefly trace how the images of teachers were conceived and have changed throughout history. Next, I will examine the political, social, and ideological influences on these images. I will then explore the implications of these images on teachers' own professional identity and willingness to incorporate reform-oriented practices in their classroom. Analysis of qualitative studies that explore these issues from the teachers' perspectives are presented. We end with a discussion about the irreconcilable tensions, silences, and a sense of becoming victims of the current blame-games in education.

CHAPTER 3

Choosing a Review Topic
and Formulating a Research Question

As you are getting ready to start your literature review, you are probably asking yourself what the next step should be in the process. As described in Chapter 2, there are several types of literature reviews, but it is generally agreed that regardless of the type of review you are writing, you should start the process by identifying the topic of your research, then narrowing it down by sharpening its focus, followed by the articulation of your research question. The topic you identify for your review and, consequently, your research question may evolve during the course of the writing process as you advance your knowledge. A better and deeper understanding of the complexities of the subject you are writing about will help you formulate a clearer and more concise question. Even though some changes and modifications may occur, starting the process by identifying a general topic and formulating a question will help you organize your literature review better and enhance its effectiveness.

In this chapter, we focus on the first stage of the review—identifying the research focus—and provide guidelines for selecting an area of interest and turning it into a topic of study. We proceed by offering strategies for narrowing down the broad topic and finding the significance it has for a wider audience. We end by formulating and refining a research question that will guide your inquiry. We also point out the differences in formulating quantitative and qualitative questions and highlight how the different types of review—systematic, traditional–narrative, and hermeneutic–phenomenological—impact the way the questions are structured. We then describe the steps and strategies recommended for selecting the literature review's topic and narrowing it down to a specific research question. We end the chapter by pointing out the characteristics of good and well-written literature review questions.

IDENTIFYING THE RESEARCH FOCUS

Selecting a Topic

We suggest starting the process by writing down a list of issues that are of interest to you. For this process to be successful, allow it to be fluid. Don't limit or question yourself, but rather let your ideas come out naturally and your imagination flow.

Now go over the list several times, taking into consideration your personal, practical, and intellectual interests. Prioritize the items on the list and narrow down their number to no more than two or three. In order to acquire initial information about the issue you are considering, you may find it helpful to use online resources such as Google or Wikipedia, or print sources such as encyclopedias. Doing so will enable you to become familiar, in general terms, with current discourse, debates, and gaps in knowledge about the issues that are of interest to you. You may also consult with friends, colleagues, and your professors, to elicit their feedback and advice.

We want to reiterate that a successful experience begins with an interest in and curiosity about an issue or a concern you feel passionate about. The more curious and excited you are about a topic, the more motivated and committed you will be to complete the project successfully. Deep interest in a topic also will help you fight possible tendencies to procrastinate and to overcome obstacles that may be caused by time constraints and professional and personal obligations. We recommend, therefore, that when possible, the topic you select for the literature review be drawn from your personal, practical, or intellectual interests (Booth, Colomb, & Williams, 2008; Maxwell, 2013).

Personal interests may emerge from your everyday life and be linked to your concerns, dreams, and hopes. Take, for example, Melinda, who is a doctoral student in psychology. Melinda, a mother of a child who is challenged by a depression disorder, joined the doctoral program initially because of her desire to know more about this disorder and about treatment options. Now that she is about to launch her dissertation work she is contemplating which topic to choose for her research and literature review. Her immediate thought is about the topic of childhood depression, which is central in her family's daily life. However, at this point, after spending several years in her doctoral program, she has come to realize that the significance of this topic extends beyond her personal world. She recognizes the potential contributions of the knowledge gained through her literature review and research for parents, psychologists, social workers, educators, and the field of psychology.

Practical interests may arise from issues of policy, programmatic changes, opportunities, or problems encountered in practice. For example, Eric, an educational leadership student, is a principal of a public middle school in an affluent suburb. Eric loves his work and is well-liked by the teachers, parents, and students, as well as board members of his school. However, he is frustrated by the increasing influence of the top-down rules and the standards-driven testing on the students' learning experience. Remembering his progressive educational theories and the social justice ideals that drove him into a career in education in the first place, Eric is contemplating whether he should lead a group of similar-minded educators. Together they will work toward opening a charter school in a low-income urban area and put these theories and ideals into practice. Nevertheless, this might be a risky career move and Eric wants to know more about the nature, strengths, and pitfalls of charter schools. Searching a topic for his master's thesis he decides to choose charter schools as the focus of his work. He hopes that by systematically reviewing the studies conducted on charter schools he will be able to make an informed decision as to whether to leave his current position to start a charter school for disadvantaged students in an economically depressed area of his city.

Intellectual interests and curiosities are the third source for choosing your literature review topic. Intellectual interests are motivated by a desire to understand in depth the theoretical perspective that undergirds the issue, and to gain deep insight into the historical and current academic discourse surrounding it. For example, April, a doctoral student in curriculum studies, is considering different topics for her research. April spent several years in Thailand and in Phoenix, Arizona, in communities serving marginalized people. Based on her own life experience and interest, April decides that she wants to understand how engaging in social change around the world transforms the lives of female educators. She wants to examine the topic through the lenses of theories on culture and power, identity formation, and feminism. April is moved by her intellectual curiosity, but at the same time she hopes that the conceptual and theoretical focus of her writing will strengthen her chances of finding a position on a university faculty.

Strauss and Corbin (1990, as cited in Maxwell, 2013) stress that the touchstone of the writer's experience is a valuable indicator of the potential success of the research endeavor. At the same time, while passion and curiosity may initially drive you to conduct your investigation on a specific topic, you should eventually move beyond it and convince your readers that your exploration matters for them. Only when a literature review topic is transformed from being meaningful to you to being useful to your readers does your study acquire academic and scholarly value (Booth et al., 2008; Galvan & Galvan, 2017; Garrard, 2014).

How to Select a Topic

The checklist in Table 3.1 summarizes the steps in the process of selecting a topic.

TABLE 3.1. Steps Involved in Selecting a Topic	
Step	✓
1. Jot down a list of issues that interest you. Don't limit or question yourself—let your ideas flow.	
2. Go over the list several times and prioritize your ideas. End with no more than two or three topics.	
3. Use Google and Wikipedia or skim encyclopedia entries for general information about the topics you are considering.	
4. Consult with friends, colleagues, and your professors and share with them the topic you are considering	
5. Choose the topic that will be at the center of your review.	

GROUP WORK

Working with a partner or a group, discuss the following:

1. Explain why you are interested in this topic.
2. Share your personal, professional, and/or intellectual interests in this particular topic.
3. Describe the information you already have found in an initial search of your topic.

Narrowing the Topic

You have identified the general topic of your literature review; nevertheless, do not rush into your literature search just yet. You do not need to find *all* of the sources available on your topic nor read every article published on the general subject you have selected. The general topic may include too much information, too many factors, and overwhelming data. A plethora of studies and theories may force you to make a choice between stretching the limits of your time and energy, or writing a superficial, "one inch deep and ten miles wide" type of review. To write a manageable, high-quality review of the literature, you need to narrow your topic down. Focusing your work around a more specific and thoughtfully formulated issue will enhance your ability to go beyond fact reporting to develop a well-organized, in-depth review of the current knowledge on your subject.

The process of narrowing down the topic involves a definition of the concepts and variables that sharpen the focus of your review (Cooper, 1988, 1998). Additionally, you may want to identify the particular perspective from which it will be studied (Machi & McEvoy, 2012).

Concepts

Concepts highlight the themes or issues contained within a broader topic. To narrow a topic to a more specific one, you need to list subtopics. These subtopics reflect facets of the general topic that are of particular interest to you. Choose one of the subtopics as the focus of your research, making sure that it is not too broad or too narrow. If the subtopic still seems too broad, you may want to narrow it further by breaking it down into additional categories and choosing one of these categories as the focus of your research. On the other hand, you may decide to combine two subtopics into one (Dawidowicz, 2010). As you choose your narrow topic, be sure to pick an issue that, from your perspective, is worth investigating because it both interests you and is considered valuable by others.

For example, let's follow the process taken by Eric, the middle school principal, who chose the topic of charter schools. Eric realizes that his initial topic is too broad and the focus of his review must be narrowed down. He jots down the following subtopics that he considers as being encompassed in the broader topic of charter schools:

1. Charter schools' curricular focus and instructional approaches
2. Accountability in charter schools
3. Charter schools' contribution to achieving equality in educating disadvantaged students
4. Advantages and disadvantages of charter schools
5. Charter schools' academic performance
6. Charter schools versus public schools
7. Charter schools' "no excuse" management approach
8. The political tension surrounding charter schools
9. Charter schools as a renewal of the promise of American education
10. Innovative practices and flexibility in charter schools

Driven by his ideals of social justice and equity and wondering whether starting a charter school would help him accomplish these goals, Eric decides to combine topics 3 and 4, which examine the strengths and pitfalls of charter schools when it comes to educating disadvantaged students. His topic, then, becomes "The Benefits and Drawbacks of Charter Schools for Disadvantaged Students." Eric shares his narrowed-down topic with his professor, who encourages him to pursue his study but suggests that the topic is still too broad and Eric should add operational variables.

Operational Variables

To delimit the topic further, you may want to use *operational variables* such as age, ethnicity/race, setting, or type of education that describe the characteristics of the population you will consider as the center of your review (Pan, 2013).

Eric agrees with his professor's advice that adding one or two operational variables will make his topic more manageable and researchable. The first operational variable he selects is the grade level of disadvantage students. The topic now reads: "The Benefits and Drawbacks of Charter Schools for Middle School Disadvantaged Students."

The second operational variable Eric selected was specific location of the schools: "The Benefits and Drawbacks of Charter Schools for Middle School Disadvantaged Students in Inner-City Districts."

Not all researchers agree about the use of operational definitions at this stage. Cooper (1998), for example, asserts that while outlining the operational definitions is useful, the writer may begin the literature review with only conceptual components and the operational variables may be added along the way.

The last step in the process of refining and narrowing the topic of the literature review is the selection of the topic's perspective.

The Topic's Perspective

The vantage point from which the literature review subject is explored indicates the author's perspective on the topic (Machi & McEvoy, 2012). For example, when discussing the strengths and weaknesses of charters school, Eric needs to decide what angle he wants to emphasize. He may choose whether he wants to highlight academic achievement expressed in standardized test scores or stress the school's social environment and its impact on students' emotional and social growth. The first perspective emphasizes organizational theory and is based largely on quantitative and measurable findings. The second perspective highlights the relational perspective and uses mostly qualitative–interpretive research. True to his personal dispositions, Eric decides to look at the latter perspective since he believes that the social–emotional environment impacts students' motivation and, consequently, their academic performance. He phrases his topic like this: The Benefits and Drawbacks of Charter School's **Social–Emotional Environment for Middle-School Disadvantaged Students in Poor Urban Districts.** At this point, Eric feels that he has narrowed down his topic sufficiently and is ready to advance to the next step.

TO DO: *Steps Involved in the Process of Narrowing Down a Topic*

Like Eric, you, too, need to narrow down your topic and transform the broad subject into a focused, researchable one. After reading the literature, you may want to revisit and further revise your narrowed-down topic. (See the checklist in Table 3.2; see also Chapter 4 for further discussions of the issue of narrowing or expanding the research topic.)

TABLE 3.2. Steps Involved in Narrowing Down a Topic	
Step	✓
1. Jot down the subtopics that are encompassed in the broad topic.	
2. Choose one of the subtopics as the center of your research. If this subtopic is still too broad, narrow it further. On the other hand, you may decide to combine two subtopics into one.	
3. List operational variables that describe the characteristics of the population you consider as the center of your review.	
4. Select a perspective—a theory, viewpoint, or research approach—from which to explore the literature.	

AUDIENCE

The last consideration in planning for your literature review is considering the audience for the review. Consider who you are writing for. If you are writing a thesis or dissertation, you may want to take into account your professor's guidelines or the expectations of your thesis or dissertation committee. If you are writing your literature review as part of a grant proposal, you should be cognizant of the criteria that will be used to evaluate your proposal. Alternatively, if the literature review is part of an article you are submitting for publication, follow the manuscript guidelines for the journals in which you would like your article to be published. In addition, it is important to keep in mind the audience that will benefit from the knowledge gained through your review. For example, are they practitioners in the field, policymakers, the general public, workplace colleagues, or members of the scholarly community?

You are now ready to present your focused topic and to articulate the rationale for limiting its scope. Your explanation also should address the significance of the topic to the readers of your study and to your professional community. Reflect on whether the topic parameters are clearly defined and whether the topic is narrow enough, or possibly too narrow.

|||||||||||||||||||||||||||||||||||||||||||||||||||||||||||||||||||||||||||||| **THE SIGNIFICANCE OF YOUR TOPIC**

There are four arguments that may highlight the significance of your study and its contribution to the field: significance for theory, significance for policy, significance for practice, and significance for social action (Marshall & Rossman, 2015).

Significance for Theory

The significance statement discusses how the study will contribute in meaningful, imaginative, and thought-provoking ways to the current discourse about the theoretical traditions and conceptual perceptions of the field. You may also highlight how the study you conduct will contribute to the extension of previous theory and refine its theoretical propositions. For example, if your study is focused on community involvement in children's education, you may discuss Urie Bronfenbrenner's (1979) theory of human ecology. In your discussion, you may point out the importance that Bronfenbrenner places on the social settings in which the school is located and its influence on students' educational, social, and emotional growth. When discussing the significance of your work, you may point out its potential contribution in expanding Bronfenbrenner's theory by including the virtual community of electronic social networks among the influencing factors.

Significance for Policy

The significance statement emphasizes how the study will contribute to overcoming problems and deficiencies in current policies related to the issue of the study. For example, you may present statistical implications of the current punitive policy for teachers and students in poverty areas whose test results are lower than expected. If your study addresses this problem, it has the potential of contributing to the school system's assessment policies and regulations.

Significance for Practice

The significance of the study may lie in finding practical solutions, articulated in the literature, to problems or concerns at the center of your study. For example, if your research topic is the challenges of reentering society after incarceration, your study may cite experts and research data that explore successful (or unsuccessful) practices of reintegration into society in vocational, housing, educational, and familial domains.

Significance for Action

Finally, a study may be significant due to its discussion of the circumstances or life experience of victims of injustice in order to motivate people to take action and bring about change in the current hurtful situation. For example, if your study focuses on the life experiences of children who were victims of sexual abuse, your literature review may explore research on these children's day-to-day experiences, their emotional vulnerability, onset of depression, and resiliency.

Your study may contribute to all four domains but not equally. In your statement you should point out which of these four is at the center of your work. For example, if the topic of your study is the enrollment of homeless children in local public schools, the significance of your research may be in the domains of theory, policy, practice, and social action. If the significance of your work lies in the domain of theory, then the emphasis of your work is on the impact of homelessness on the identity and social–psychological development of children. If your review highlights the significance of policy, then your focus may be on local, state, and national regulations and laws involved in enrolling homeless children in school. If, on the other hand, at the center of your review are ways of enhancing homeless children's academic and social growth, then the significance of your research is in the practice domain. The social action significance of your work is highlighted when you spotlight the unjust experiences of homeless children and advocate for social actions to improve these conditions. All of these studies have significant contributions to the field, but as a writer you need to decide which of the four is most important for you. This choice has clear implications for the research question you will formulate and for the literature you will review.

We realize that at this point of the review-writing process, as you are choosing your topic and formulating your research question, you may not be ready to fully express the significance of work. Nevertheless, it is important that you start thinking about it and considering your study's potential contributions to the field and its meaning to your audience.

Table 3.3 highlights the questions that will help you identify the audience for your study and determine its significance.

TABLE 3.3. Identifying the Audience for the Study and Its Significance	
Questions to ask	**Explain**
1. Who is the audience of your study?	
2. Is your study significant for theory?	
3. Is your study significant for policy?	
4. Is your study significant for practice?	
5. Is your study significant for social action?	

GROUP WORK

Working with a partner or a group, discuss the following:

1. What subtopics of your more general topic are of interest to you?
2. Why did you choose this aspect of the general topic as the center of your research?
3. What are the operational variables that describe the population you want to study?
4. What perspective will you use to explore the literature?
5. Who is your intended audience? How will this choice impact your writing?
6. What is the significance of your work to the field? Be as specific as possible.

THE RESEARCH QUESTION

Formulating the Research Questions

Once you have set the parameters of your topic and specified its scope, you are ready to formulate your research question. This question will guide you in searching the current literature on your topic. It will also shape how you read and analyze these sources and how you construct and write your review.

Research questions may have several purposes. According to Booth et al. (2008), the research question often aims to:

> ► extend the current knowledge
> ► close a gap in the current knowledge
> ► support existing knowledge with new evidence
> ► explore theoretical perspective(s) that underlie the topic
> ► solve a problem
> ► open the topic to different research approaches or lines of investigation
> ► disagree, contradict, or point out inconsistencies in current research

Research questions reflect (1) the types of approaches to research and (2) the kinds of literature review being undertaken. The following is a discussion of these points.

Research Questions According to the Approach to Research

Before you phrase your literature review question, you may want to go back and review the three approaches to research that were discussed in Chapter 2: quantitative, qualitative, and mixed methods. This will allow you to decide which lens to use in formulating your research question. The following is a brief description of what distinguishes quantitative, qualitative, and mixed-methods questions.

Quantitative questions are stated in a way that directs the writer to assess outcomes, measure consequences, and statistically compare relationships between different variables as well as differences between groups. Thus, these questions may be designed to assess the outcomes and effects of a particular practice, treatment, program, or policy. For example, Melinda, the doctoral student who wants to explore the topic of depression among children, may focus her question on the measurable results of specific group treatment interventions on children's social interactions. She may phrase it as "What are the different effects of three small group therapy approaches on the level of social interactions with peers of children with depression?"

Qualitative questions are stated in an open-ended style, often using "how" and "what" questions. This style of question emphasizes *processes* and how they are experienced from the perspective of individuals or groups. The question may also highlight the contexts in which particular practices, programs, or policies are implemented. For example, Melinda could phrase her literature review question as "How do children with depression who participated in group therapy perceive their social interactions with their peers?"

Mixed-methods questions are a third option for you to consider. Choosing this style allows you to combine questions that focus on statistical, measurable outcomes, as well as on the personal experiences of those involved. For example, as a third choice for her literature review question, Melinda might state the following: "What are the effects of group therapy on children with depression and how do they experience their social relationships with their peers"?

Research Questions According to the Kind of Literature Review

The kind of question you are posing for your literature review and the way you formulate your question are also influenced by the style of literature review you have chosen to write. The following is a brief description of the characteristics of questions for systematic, traditional–narrative, and hermeneutic–phenomenological reviews.

Systematic Review

In a systematic review it is critical that the research questions be precisely defined. This question determines the decisions the writer makes about what studies to include or exclude from the review. To ensure that the decisions are objective and consistent, each concept within the questions, should be carefully defined (Jesson et al., 2011).

The questions used for systematic reviews are mostly quantitative in nature and should be stated using clear selection criteria. Higgins and Green (2011) suggest that the questions be formulated around the following specifications:

1. The type of **population** targeted, including characteristics such as age, gender, socioeconomic status, and occupation.

2. The type of **intervention** used, such as action, program, treatment, or policy.

3. The type of **research design** used to carry out the investigation, such as experimental or descriptive.

4. The type of **outcomes** and how they are measured, such as test scores and behavior observations.

5. The type of **context** in which the research questions are studied, such as setting and circumstances.

The following is an example of a question in a systematic review:

What are the changes between the beginning and end-of-year knowledge and skills of first-year social work students as a result of an intense mentoring program?

In this example, the population comprises first-year social work students; the intervention is an intensive mentoring program; the research design is experimental (changes from beginning to end-of-year scores); the outcomes are knowledge and skills; and the context is social work training.

The systematic review questions should be finalized before the search for literature sources begins. Any change in the way the original question is phrased, as well as any selection of references that does not match the original question, is strongly discouraged. Such changes are perceived as compromising the validity of the review's conclusions.

Traditional–Narrative Review

According to a traditional–narrative review, the research question should be narrowed down but still be broad enough to incorporate different research approaches and methods. The emphasis is mostly on studies with qualitative and mixed-methods research. In addition, you may consider the theories, concepts, or issues contained in your topic, the variables that are important, and the perspective you want to highlight.

It is acceptable for the initial research question to evolve and be refined as the literature review process advances. To illustrate the way traditional–narrative research questions are usually phrased, we present the same example of mentoring first-year social workers used above.

How does the experience of mentoring influence first-year social workers' perceptions of their profession and their work job satisfaction?

As you notice, the question is open-ended and does not include the specific criteria as was the case in a systematic review.

Hermeneutic–Phenomenological Review

For a hermeneutic–phenomenological review author, it is obvious that the particular research question cannot be completely identified until the writer is deeply engaged in the review process. Only when the researcher is immersed in the readings, and the ideas emerge through interactions with different sources, does the research question reveal itself. Still, we recommend that if your literature review follows this approach, start the review cycle by posing a broad, open-ended question that states the intended focus of your review. This preliminary question is often based on your previous readings or life experience. This, in turn, will probably result in refining or even changing your preliminary question. Thus, the refinement of the initial question goes hand in hand with the process of reading (Boell & Cecez-Kecmanovic, 2010, 2014).

For example, let's illustrate the nature of a research question in a hermeneutic–phenomenological review using the same topic of mentoring first-year social workers that was mentioned above. The question may be as follows:

What is the role of relationships in forming social workers' view of self and how is it affected by the mentoring relationship?

This example of a hermeneutic–phenomenological question is open ended, and is mostly focused on concepts, relationships, and perceptions.

Writing the Research Question

Now that we have considered the different types of research questions that reflect the type of research and the kinds of review you plan to conduct and the influence of those on the way the question is framed, you are ready to write your own research question. As you write your question, contemplate what you want to achieve. For example, do you want to close the gap in current knowledge, extend current research, or solve a problem?

You may want to write several questions on your topic or perhaps several versions of the same question. Read and reread what you have written and choose the one that sparks your interest most. Evaluate the way the question was phrased according to the types of research questions outlined above and, if needed, revise or polish the phrasing.

You may find it helpful to assess the research questions with the help of your group or learning partner. In your discussion, make sure to consider the characteristics that define good research questions, as well as what needs to be avoided.

To formulate your research question, you may want to follow the steps in Table 3.4.

Steps Involved in Formulating the Research Question

Table 3.4 provides a list of steps for formulating your research question.

TABLE 3.4. Steps Involved in Formulating the Research Question
Step
1. Decide whether your question will be framed as a quantitative, qualitative, or a mixed-methods question.
2. Formulate the question according to the type of review you are conducting: systematic, traditional–narrative, or hermeneutic–phenomenological.
3. Consider what you are aiming to achieve with your question.
4. Write several versions of your research question and choose the one that can help you attain your review goals.
5. Choose the topic that will be at the center of your review.

What Is a Good Question?

As you assess your question individually or with a group member, consider the following characteristics that distinguish good research questions, as well as what needs to be avoided:

A good research question is:

▶ meaningful and worth investigating. Your question should have a personal, practical, and/or theoretical meaning to you, but it also should have significance for others in your field.

▶ phrased concisely and should be clear to you and your readers.

▶ not too broad, but rather manageable and doable in the allotted time. On the other hand, a good research question should not be too narrow, thereby making your review too limited and lacking depth.

▶ framed in a way that will guide the literature search.

▶ phrased in a way that includes at least some of the key terms that can be used for the literature search.

▶ answerable through a process of reading, analyzing, and synthesizing the relevant literature on the topic. A question like "How will the use of graphic novels in middle school classes impact the vocabulary of future high school students?" is interesting but unanswerable since we can't research now what will happen in the future. A better question might be "What are the influences of graphic novels on young adults' motivation to read?"

▶ phrased in a way that allows for different approaches or outcomes and does not dictate one answer (such as yes/no answers).

▶ not formed on questionable or unproven presuppositions. For example, the question "How will hypnosis, which helps overcome insecurities, impact people's fear of public speaking?" is based on an unproven premise that hypnosis helps people overcome fear of public speaking.

▶ not stated as a factual question that can be answered easily through an informal search (e.g., by using Google or Wikipedia). For example, an answer to a question like "What are the state laws for suspending students on the basis of their behavior?" can be easily found through an Internet search. A better question would be "How does the implementation of state suspension laws impact high school students' behavior in school?"

GROUP WORK

In your literature review group, introduce your question and your chosen style of review, and discuss the following with your peers:

1. Is the question clear?

2. Does the question achieve your goals? Do you want to close the gap in current knowledge, extend current research, or solve a problem?

3. Are the concepts and key variables in the question clearly articulated? What are the keywords (search terms) in the question that will help you conduct the library search?

PREPLANNING THE LIBRARY SEARCH ||||||||||||||||||||||||||||||||||||||||||||||||||||||||||||||||||||||||||||

In Chapter 4 we focus on the specific steps in conducting a literature search. The steps described in that chapter can be used for gathering information in different types of literature review. Here we highlight some points for you to consider prior to starting your library search. In these points, we explain how you may adjust the search based on the type of literature review you plan to conduct. These types include systematic, traditional–narrative, and hermeneutic–phenomenological reviews. In describing each type, we also present tables that may assist with your selection of sources.

Systematic Review

Systematic review writers recommend using specific and detailed criteria for selecting sources. These criteria become a part of the literature review. Table 3.5 (p. 53) illustrates typical criteria for such a review. We recommend that you begin filling in the table by stating your research question.

TABLE 3.5. Criteria for Selecting Sources for a Systematic Review	
Research question	
Target population	
Intervention examined	
Study design	
Outcome	
Context	

In addition, in order to protect the objectivity and scientific nature of your systematic review, it is recommended that you develop a protocol that specifies the research terms, the title of database used, the dates that the library search was conducted, the years covered, the language restrictions, and the number of hits (Table 3.6). As before, start completing the table by stating your question.

TABLE 3.6. Protocol for a Systematic Literature Search	
Review question	
Search terms	
Database title	
Dates of conducting the search	
Years covered	
Language restriction	
Number of hits	

Traditional–Narrative Review

Articulating the criteria for the library search is not required for the traditional–narrative style of review. Nevertheless, we still recommend that the criteria for your library search be stated in the introduction to your review. We also suggest that you briefly note the process of your search. Table 3.7 illustrates some of the items that may be included in your description.

Hermeneutic–Phenomenological Review

The initial search for a hermeneutical–phenomenological literature review reflects the writers' previous readings and their preconceived notions about the topic. Their reading of one source often leads to their next choice of books or articles as their understanding about the phenomenon expands and their knowledge about the seminal authors writing about the topic grows. In the introduction to the literature review, the writers' choice of literature and their discussion about their choices often highlight their subjectivity, which is drawn from their life experience. Table 3.8 (p. 55) shows some of the items that may be included in a literature search for a hermeneutic–phenomenological review.

TABLE 3.7. Criteria for Selecting Sources for a Traditional–Narrative Review	
Review question	
Search terms	
Research approach and methods	
Theory (theories) undergirding the topic	
Concepts at the center of the review	
Variables	
The perspectives you want to highlight	

TABLE 3.8. Literature Search for a Hermeneutic–Phenomenological Review	
Initial review questions	
Personal background that shaped the research questions choice	
Preconceived notions about the research questions	
Readings that influenced the research question choice	
Main authors and thinkers on the literature search list	
Keywords (search terms) that may initiate the library search	

WHAT'S NEXT?

In this chapter we focused on the process of turning an area of interest into your topic of study, considering its significance, and formulating the research question(s) that will guide your inquiry. We provided suggestions for preplanning the library research and offer criteria for selecting sources. In the next chapter, we describe strategies and techniques for locating sources through traditional and digital libraries and other online databases.

CHAPTER SUMMARY

1. You should start your literature review by identifying a research topic that is meaningful to you and doable, with potential contributions to the field.

2. After identifying your topic of interest, the next step is to narrow it to avoid the need to collect an overwhelming amount of data. This process involves defining concepts, variables, and the particular perspective from which you will study the topic.

3. When discussing the focus of the literature review, you should consider the audience of the study and highlight the significance of your study and its potential contribution to the field.

4. Research questions are designed to address issues such as extending current knowledge, closing gaps in knowledge, supporting existing knowledge with new evidence, solving a problem, using different approaches to study previously investigated topics, and supporting or pointing out inconsistencies or deficiencies in previous research.

5. Research questions are reflective of the three approaches to research (quantitative, qualitative, and mixed methods) and the kinds of literature review being undertaken (systematic, traditional–narrative, and hermeneutic–phenomenological).

6. In a systematic review, it is critical that the research questions be precisely defined. These questions should be finalized prior to undertaking the literature search.

7. In a traditional–narrative review, the research questions are broad enough to incorporate different research approaches and methods. These questions may evolve as the literature review process progresses.

8. The research question in a hermeneutic–phenomenological review may change as the writer becomes deeply engaged in the reviewing process.

9. The characteristics of a good research question include the following: It is meaningful; it is phrased precisely and clearly; it is not too broad or too narrow; it guides the literature search; it includes at least some key search terms; it does not call for yes/no answers; it is not based on unproven or questionable presuppositions; and it does not call for merely factual information that be found through a superficial search.

10. It is recommended that the criteria for library research be discussed in the introduction to traditional–narrative literature reviews, whereas including such criteria is required for systematic reviews. In hermeneutic–phenomenological reviews, writers reflect on the subjectivity of their literature choices.

IIIIIIIIIIIIIIIIIIIIIIIIIIIIIIIIIIIIIIIIIIIIIIIIIIIIIIIIIIIIICHAPTER 4

Locating and Organizing Research Sources

At this point, you have selected your topic, considered its significance, and formulated your research question. As we discussed in Chapter 3, your question may evolve and change as you immerse yourself in the reading process. Now you are ready to search for appropriate articles, books, reports, and other sources that will serve as the basis for your literature review. This search should be a systematic, meticulous, careful, and thoughtful process. Searching the literature can start with an initial, general idea about your topic of interest, continue when you sharpen the focus of your study, and conclude when you finalize writing the literature review.

In this chapter we discuss what a literature search is and explain its purposes. We differentiate between primary, secondary, and tertiary sources and consider the kinds of references you should look for. We outline the techniques and strategies for finding sources through traditional and digital libraries and other online databases. We end the chapter by suggesting how you can track and record your search and the sources you have obtained, and offer ways for you to start to create your bibliography.

Figure 4.1 (p. 58) illustrates the process of searching for information on your topic. Although we describe the search process as linear and sequential, in practice it is ongoing and may continue while you write the literature review, conduct the research study, or even write the final report (Hart, 2001). Based on the information you collect throughout the search, you may modify, refine, or even change the topic you want to investigate for your literature review.

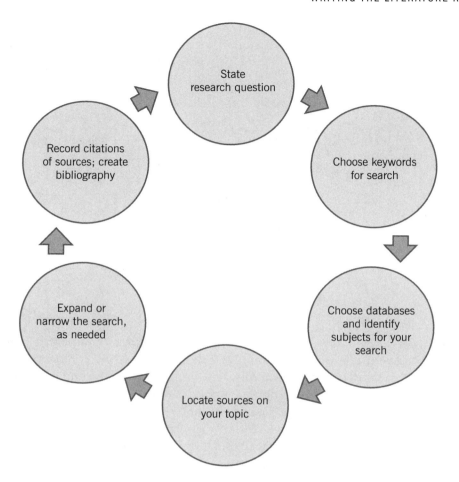

FIGURE 4.1. A diagram of the library search process.

THE PURPOSE OF SEARCHING THE LITERATURE ||||||||||||||||||||||||||||||||||||||||||||||||||||||||||||||||||||

Searching the literature is an essential step in the process of conducting a literature review. Without a purposeful and effective search of the literature, your study "may lack the breadth and depth of understanding expected for your level and type of project" (Hart, 2001, p. 8). Conducting a literature search will allow you to:

1. Gather background information and become more knowledgeable about your topic. This will help you sharpen the focus of your study and zero in on the exact topic you want to investigate.

2. Identify publications that are centered on your particular field of interest to allow you to move from general to more focused sources.

3. Decide whether you need to expand or narrow down your search based on the number of sources you find. This is especially true when you are either inundated with sources or fear that you may be missing important literature about your topic.

4. Avoid presenting a biased or shallow description of the current knowledge regarding the topic you are researching. A good search allows you to become familiar with different points of view, perspectives, and theories concerning your area of interest.

SOURCE MATERIALS FOR THE LITERATURE REVIEW

There are different types of materials available to researchers seeking to find information about their topic. While printed materials used to be the standard years ago, today's search engines enable researchers to locate more information electronically and to do so faster and more efficiently. However, the quality and trustworthiness of the information found online has to be established and confirmed. In the days of print information, the main sources were books and journal articles; conference papers were available in microfiche. Though it may have been harder to locate such sources, once you found them, you could be confident that they were submitted for peer review and were vetted by experts in the field. With the explosion of the Internet and electronic search engines, the availability of references and other documents and information is no longer an issue. At the same time, information found on the Internet is not always submitted for peer review, and quality control may not be exercised prior to its being shared with the general public. Thus, although search engines are excellent tools for gathering information about your topic, you have to establish its reliability, validity, and trustworthiness.

There are several types of source materials, including books, articles, conference papers, and reviews. There is also what is referred to as "gray literature," defined as publications that are not disseminated for commercial purposes. These include dissertations, "white papers," monographs, and government reports. Sources can also be classified by dividing them into *primary*, *secondary*, and *tertiary*. The definition and examples of each type of source may vary depending on the discipline and field where they are used. Education, humanities, and social research often use the following descriptions for each type of source.

Primary sources are firsthand accounts and reports written by the researchers who conducted the study, and they offer an insider's view. Examples of primary sources include field notes, research reports, articles written by the researchers, lab reports, artifacts, diaries, autobiographies, interviews, videos, audio recordings, meeting minutes, and proceeding recordings. Due to the increasing ease of digitalizing various forms of primary sources, they are more readily available to researchers looking for information about their topic of interest.

Secondary sources are summaries, discussions, and interpretations of primary original-work sources that were previously presented elsewhere. Examples of secondary sources are journal articles or reports that summarize, report on, or critique other researchers' work; biographies; and commentaries. Summaries or evaluations of events that happened in the past are also considered secondary sources. The authors of secondary sources do not have firsthand experience, but they have a richer and often less biased perspective compared with that of the primary-source writers.

Tertiary sources are those that summarize and critically evaluate and review primary and secondary research sources. Examples of tertiary sources are encyclopedias (including Wikipedia), textbooks, bibliographies, almanacs, indexes, guidebooks, handbooks, and manuals. Sources classified as tertiary by some people or disciplines may be considered secondary by others. For example, in some disciplines textbooks are considered secondary sources while in others they are referred to as tertiary.

Table 4.1 compares primary, secondary, and tertiary sources, pointing out their advantages and disadvantages.

TABLE 4.1. A Comparison of Primary, Secondary, and Tertiary Sources

Source	Description	Advantages	Disadvantages
Primary sources	■ Firsthand experiences and reports written by researchers who conducted the studies	■ Offer insider view ■ Provide firsthand experience	■ May be biased ■ At times are harder to obtain
Secondary sources	■ Summaries, discussions, and interpretations of primary original-work sources that were previously presented elsewhere	■ Likely to have a less biased perspective ■ Often a summary of multiple sources and perspectives around certain aspects of the topic ■ Provide a focused analysis of the subject of interest	■ Authors do not have firsthand experience with the particular research
Tertiary sources	■ Summaries and critical evaluation of primary as well as secondary research sources	■ Holistic ■ Summarize and evaluate multiple sources ■ Provide an introduction to the main leaders, main theories, and "big ideas" in the field	■ Lack firsthand experience with the particular study ■ Less in-depth description of each individual study

"WORKING BACKWARDS" SEARCH

Many experienced researchers recommend that you start by reading tertiary sources that summarize your topic, provide references and bibliographies, and list primary and secondary sources. Additionally, tertiary sources provide a holistic picture and the context of a topic, as well as an initial understanding of the main theories and leaders in the field. Your next step should be consulting secondary sources that describe the state of research on your topic and provide a more focused analysis of your subject of interest. These sources may also highlight where additional research is needed and provide ideas for the methodology that you could use for your study. After you gain a good understanding of the main issues related to your topic, you then move on to the final step of finding primary sources. At this point you possess the proper tools to assess and appreciate primary sources that describe the direct, firsthand experiences of researchers in the field.

LOCATING YOUR LITERATURE REVIEW SOURCES

The process of searching the literature can be overwhelming due to the constantly growing number of databases and search engines. Generally, with the exception of a systematic review, the literature review can be seen as a treasure hunt: each reference you find leads you to additional studies. This process is also referred to as a *snowball effect* that allows you to continue to gather additional references that are cited in those you already have, thus expanding and multiplying your sources. Therefore, when searching for sources on your topic, it is always a good idea to start with the most recent research you can find because it will include an updated literature review and references on your topic.

One of your first steps should probably be an initial exploratory online search on your topic and a visit to your library. Librarians are an invaluable source of information and guidance, especially considering the fast pace of changes in information retrieval systems. As stated by broadcaster and journalist Linton Weeks, "In the nonstop tsunami of global information, librarians provide us with floaties and teach us to swim" (*www.goodreads.com/author/quotes/1498146.Linton_Weeks*).

To assist novice researchers, most college libraries have posted on their website modules and guidebooks describing the search process. You may check your library website to determine if such information is available. If you are on campus, you may want to schedule a one-on-one meeting with a librarian to get you started. Public libraries are also an excellent source, and a scheduled meeting with their reference librarian can steer you in the right direction.

Throughout the process of your search, remember to record carefully, meticulously, and systematically every source that you find to enable you to retrieve this information more easily when needed. Later in this chapter we offer suggestions on how to record and summarize the references that you gather.

Searching Electronic Databases

Searching electronic databases is an efficient process that can provide a great number of sources in a short amount of time. In order for your search to be effective, you have to use the most accurate *keywords* or search terms that relate to your research topic. When you enter the chosen keywords into search boxes to obtain sources on your subject, all the searchable fields in the records (such as titles, abstracts, and the author's name) are searched. Using a variety of synonyms for the keywords can improve your search results because different authors use different terminology for the same terms.

Looking at your research questions, you may be able to condense or represent the issue they entail using a few short terms. For example, your research question may deal with the best techniques and approaches to enhance vocabulary development in preschool children. You can choose terms such as "language development," "speech development," or "vocabulary development." Search terms such as "early childhood" or "preschool children" could be used to find articles that focus on the specific age range of the children for your research. In another research question example, the question may center on the differences in the way men and women communicate. Phrases such as "interpersonal communication" and "gender differences" reflect the keywords of your research question. Also note that adding quotation marks to the words causes the database to search for these words as a phrase.

Another way to search databases and library catalogs is to use a *subject* or *descriptor.* (Depending on the discipline, one of these two terms may be used. For example, the ERIC database uses the term *descriptor.*) A subject is a specific term used to categorize the source. Subjects are assigned as access points by the author of the article, by the database, or by the library catalog to describe the content of items in a database. The subject is a controlled term used by the discipline, and therefore it is less flexible and is more likely to yield fewer sources compared with a search using keywords. On the other hand, using subjects allows for a more focused search that produces results more relevant to your topic.

Another difference between keywords and subjects is that keywords can be searched for anywhere in the searchable records whereas subjects can be searched for only in the designated field for the record. For example, if you search for the subject "immigration" and the word appeared in the article title but not in the subject field, the article will not be retrieved in your search results. If you search for the keyword "immigration," the word could appear in any of the fields that are being searched by the database and the article will appear in your search results.

Make sure you spell out all acronyms when conducting your search to ensure that you obtain as many relevant sources on your topic as possible. For example, when searching for articles on STEM (science, technology, engineering, and math), using the acronym only, you will get articles on stem cell research, stem cell engineering, and stem cell biology.

Table 4.2 includes a brief description of keywords (search words) and subjects (descriptors), as well as their advantages and disadvantages.

At times, a good article on your topic may serve as a valuable source for identifying other keywords or subjects listed for that article. This may lead you to consider new search terms that you did not use before

Another helpful source for locating keywords is a thesaurus, which is a dictionary containing a systematic list of synonyms and related words that have similar meanings; sometimes antonyms are also included. Many disciplines have their own thesaurus that allow you to find discipline-specific terms. For example, George, a doctoral student in social work, is searching the term "resilience." His ERIC search (*http://eric.ed.gov*) shows how the term is defined under Scope Note and the category that it appears under, as well as other related terms (see Figure 4.2, p. 64). George can use this information to refine his search and to find additional useful sources through the use of related terms.

It is important to use appropriate search terms. A thesaurus can help you identify such terms if your initial search does not yield a sufficient number of relevant sources. For example, suppose your topic relates to stealing intellectual property. Using the ERIC database, operated by the U.S. Department of Education (*http://eric.ed.gov*), you type in your search box the words "intellectual theft." The search yields no hits on the topic. Using the ERIC thesaurus (*http://eric.ed.gov/?ti=I*), browse and scroll down to the word *intellectual*. One of the choices is *intellectual property*. Note that the information provided by ERIC also includes a broader term (*ownership*), a narrower term (*copyright*), and related terms that you can use for your search (e.g., *plagiarism*).

TABLE 4.2. Comparing and Contrasting Keywords and Subjects

Keywords	vs. Subjects
■ natural language words describing your topic—good to start with	■ predefined "controlled vocabulary" words used to describe the content of each item (book, journal article) in a database
■ more flexible to search by—can combine together in many ways	■ less flexible to search by—need to know the exact controlled vocabulary term
■ database looks for keywords anywhere in the record—not necessarily connected together	■ database looks for subjects only in the subject heading or descriptor field, where the most relevant words appear
■ may yield too many or too few results	■ if too many results, also uses subheadings to focus on one aspect of the broader subject
■ may yield many irrelevant results	■ results usually very relevant to the topic

Source: MIT Libraries (*https://libguides.mit.edu/c.php?g=175963&p=1160804*).

Resilience (Psychology)

Scope Note: The capacity of individuals to withstand, cope with, or recover from adverse, stressful, or high-risk circumstances. Protective factors that enhance this ability may be internal (personal attributes such as self-efficacy, spirituality, etc.) or external (e.g., relationships such as supportive family or community ties). From 2004 to 2010, this concept was indexed with the descriptor "Personality Traits." Prior to 2004, the concept may have been indexed with the identifiers "Ego Resilience," "Career Resilience," "Resilience (Career)," and "Resilience (Ego)."

Category: Individual Development and Characteristics

Search collection using this descriptor	
Use this term instead of Resilience (Academic) Resilience (Personality) (2004)	Related Terms Adjustment (to Environment) At-Risk Students Coping Goal Orientation Persistence Self-Esteem Self-Management Social Support Groups Stress Management Student Attitudes Student Characteristics

FIGURE 4.2. Screen shot of George's ERIC search of the keyword "resilience."

Using ERIC, you can search by thesaurus descriptors (i.e., subjects) that are organized alphabetically. The ERIC database will look for your search terms across a set of key ERIC fields. These fields are title, author, source, abstract, and descriptor. The results are sorted in categories such as publication date, descriptor, source, author, publication type, education level, and audience.

Most disciplines have databases that can be searched electronically. For example, in addition to the ERIC database, the EBSCO system (*www.ebscohost.com*) offers library resources to customers in academic, medical, K–12, public library, law, corporate, and government markets. (Researchers who are not accessing ERIC or EBSCO through their institutions can use the free site at *http://eric.ed.gov*).

Examples of other databases include: PsycINFO (*www.apa.org/pubs/databases/psycinfo/index.aspx*), which is offered by the American Psychological Association; a variety of EBSCO databases (*www.ebscohost.com*) in the humanities and social sciences; and ProQuest (*www.proquest.com*), which covers multiple subjects and offers services to students. Elsevier, which includes Scopus (*www.elsevier.com/solutions/scopus*), is a commercially available database that provides abstracts and a citation database of peer-reviewed literature in the areas of science, technology, medicine, social sciences, arts, and humanities. Due to membership restrictions, you should check with your local library to determine what databases it subscribes to and then run your own search using those databases.

Additionally, search engines such as Google Scholar (*http://scholar.google.com*) are readily available to the general public. Google Scholar is limited to scholarly sources, and it filters out popular and commercial sources that are not scholarly. Full text may not always be available via Google Scholar, but often libraries can obtain these sources through interlibrary loan. Additionally, to uncover books on your topic, you can try searching websites such as Amazon (*www.amazon.com*).

While most universities do not accept Wikipedia (*www.wikipedia.org*) as a reference in academic work, you may use it to get a general introduction to your topic (Ridley, 2012). Keep in mind, though, that the sources being cited and the information provided in Wikipedia were not vetted by experts.

You may also want to consider using other, more general online resources that are widely available. Various professional organizations maintain websites, as do governments and other groups. You will recognize these resources by their website addresses that are likely to end with *.gov* or *.org*. For example, the U.S. Department of Education (*www.ed.gov*) maintains a website that includes information on education data and research (e.g., National Center for Education Statistics, What Works Clearinghouse, and the Nation's Report Card). The ERIC database allows users to search for information by publication date, full text only, and peer reviewed.

 How to Locate Your Literature Sources

Table 4.3 provides a checklist for locating your library sources.

TABLE 4.3. Locating Your Literature Review Sources	
Step	✓
1. Start with the most recent research you can find on your topic.	
2. Do an exploratory online search on your topic at home or in the library.	
3. Record carefully and systematically throughout the process every source you find to enable you to retrieve this information more easily later.	
4. Use your research questions to find keywords, or search terms that relate to your research topic.	
5. Use a thesaurus to locate subjects/descriptors.	
6. Check out the subjects/descriptors listed for good articles you have located to consider additional search terms.	
7. Conduct an Internet search using discipline-related databases as well as readily available search engines such as Google Scholar.	

Expanding or Narrowing Your Search

When searching the literature, you may find at times that you need to expand or narrow the number of your sources. The need to expand may arise when you do not find a sufficient number of references to write an in-depth and rigorous review. On the other hand, you may need to reduce the number of sources when the search yields too many references, some of which may not be relevant to your own particular topic. Another way to focus your search is to use the Boolean operators (or connectors) OR, AND, and NOT. These operators allow you expand or narrow your research. Following are some strategies you may use if you realize that you have too few or too many relevant sources on your topic.

Expanding the Search

At times, you may decide to expand the search if you want to ensure that you cover the topic in depth, feel that you do not have a sufficient number of sources, or are afraid that you might be missing important literature on your topic. One way to expand your search is to use the operator OR, which will result in the search engine looking for sources that include two keywords. In other words, the search engine will look for sources that include either one, two, or both keywords. This will expand the search considerably. For example, Natasha, who is an assistant superintendent, writes a grant proposal for implementing nutrition education in the district and wants to document the effects of such programs on students' lunch choices. As she prepares the proposal's literature review, she is searching a database using two keywords: "nutrition education" and "school lunch program." To expand her search she is using the connector OR (see Figure 4.3).

To illustrate the process of expanding the search, let's look at Michael, a doctoral student in sociology. Michael cares deeply about issues related to the

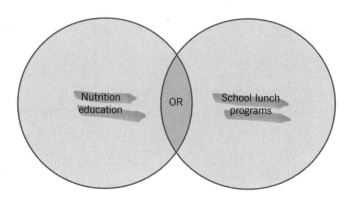

FIGURE 4.3. Using the connector OR to expand the search: The search will include both terms: "Nutrition education" and "School lunch programs."

environment and pollution, especially when it comes to urban inner-city areas, like the neighborhood where he resides. He is passionate about the importance of teaching children, starting at a young age, that guarding the environment is essential. Discussing this issue with his daughter's preschool teacher, he found to his surprise how little is done about it in her school. The teacher says that she would love to teach her students about recycling; however, she has not found any age-appropriate curriculum developed for inner-city schools. Michael and the teacher agreed that they are going to do that. Before starting their endeavor, Michael conducts a search on recycling education in inner-city preschools. Table 4.4 shows various search terms used by Michael and the number of references listed for each one.

You can also expand your search by using your keywords in a truncated form. Often, this is done by adding an asterisk (*) to the truncated search word. This is also referred to as a *wildcard*. For example, if you are interested in the subject of performing arts, the truncated search word "perform*" may generate references for topics such as performance, performing, and performer. Various databases may have other rules or suggestions for advanced searches, so you should check the databases you use carefully or consult your librarian.

Limiting the Search

Using AND will *limit* your search by requesting the search engine to look for sources that include *two* terms, either in the title or in the article itself. For example, you may recall George, the social work doctoral student mentioned above, who wants to study resilience among children in foster care. Using a database, he is searching both terms—*resilience* and *children in foster care*—by connecting them with the operator AND (Figure 4.4, p. 68). This search will limit the sources by filtering out any source that does not directly relate to his chosen topic.

A search can also be narrowed by using the connector NOT. You use this connector to specify that the second term should not appear in the search. For example, Marie, a professor at a local community college, is asked to develop

TABLE 4.4. Results of Michael's Search: Numbers of References Found under Each Search Term	
Term searched	**Number of sources**
recycling education in inner-city preschool	31
curriculum in recycling education for preschool children	32
recycling education in preschool	149
recycling education in inner-city schools	1,016
recycling education in school	4,057

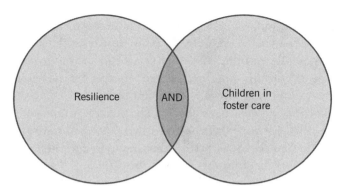

FIGURE 4.4. Using the Boolean operator AND to locate sources that relate to resilience of children in foster care, excluding other groups.

programs for adults who are learning English as a second language. As part of her proposal, she is writing a literature review on this topic. In order to exclude studies of English as a second language that were conducted with PreK–12 students rather than with adults, Marie is using the connector NOT (Figure 4.5).

Other ways to arrive at a manageable number of sources is to sharpen the focus by continuing to add descriptors that more accurately reflect the writer's topic of interest. Let's look at Anita, a history student, who decides to conduct a search of the topic of ancient Greece. Remembering that when she was a young child, her father used to read stories to her from Greek mythology, Anita decides to research the topic of ancient Greece. Her search of the term "ancient Greece" yields a huge number of sources (over 60,000). Since she is also interested in women's issues, she decides to put together her two topics of interest and focus on women in ancient Greece. The search of these two terms combined generates a smaller

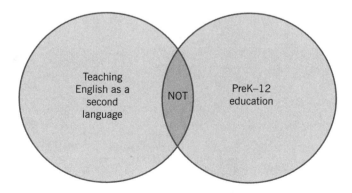

FIGURE 4.5. Using the connector NOT to search for teaching English as a second language to adults only, excluding PreK–12 learners.

number of sources (over 4,300). Anita determines that the number of sources is still too high, and therefore she narrows the topic further, focusing on the role of women in ancient Greek politics. This search produces a more manageable number of sources (over 560), although she deems it to be still too high. At this point, Anita has several options: she can further narrow her search by choosing a specific region or town in Greece, a certain time period, or certain roles in politics. She can further narrow her search by limiting it to full-text publications or sources that are available in her library system, although this step is recommended only if you are facing a short deadline.

The type of sources you want (e.g., books, articles, conference papers), the dates of publication (e.g., choosing only more current publications), the type of documents (e.g., full text), and whether they are peer reviewed can also help you focus your search and make it more manageable. Keep in mind that the choice of sources may also depend on the guidelines provided by your instructors or the grant.

If you still can't find the information you are looking for, check that you used the right terms and spelled them correctly. Ensure that your search term is not too long because it is possible that your search is designed to retrieve only sources that include the complete term. Conversely, if you use too few words your search may yield too many sources, with some of them unrelated to your topic.

TO DO: How to Expand or Narrow the Search

The checklist in Table 4.5 may assist you in expanding or narrowing your search.

TABLE 4.5. Expanding or Narrowing the Search	
Step	✓
1. Expand the search when you do not find a sufficient number of references.	
2. Narrow the search when it yields too many references or those that are not relevant to your topic.	
3. Use the connector OR to expand the search.	
4. Expand the search by using a truncated form of your keywords.	
5. Narrow the search by using the connectors AND and NOT.	
6. Sharpen the focus of your search by adding subjects/descriptors that more clearly define your topic.	
7. Choose the types of sources you want (e.g., books or articles, publication dates).	
8. Ensure that you spelled all the search terms correctly and that they are not too long or too short.	

GROUP WORK

Report to your group members on the process you have gone through in searching for sources. Describe some of the challenges, surprises, frustrations, or rewarding moments you have experienced. You may want to provide a written description of the process that you will then include in the introduction to your literature review. Box 4.1 may be helpful to you in writing this description.

RECORDING ELECTRONIC DATA SEARCH RESULTS

Most electronic databases (such as ERIC, PsycINFO, or other databases available through EBSCO) include a feature that allows you to save and mail yourself the documents that you found. You can also get the complete citations through these services. Articles that you wish to obtain but are not available full text can be requested and sent to you electronically through the services of your library. Students who are working on a literature review that is part of a thesis or dissertation may find full-text dissertations available through ProQuest (*www.proquest.com*) to be especially useful.

BOX 4.1. An Example of a Literature Search

The authors examined the literature using EBSCOHost and Premier Academic Elite. We also used the Internet to conduct a search of the *International Journal of Mentoring and Coaching in Education*, since we consider this among the leading journals in the field and, as a relatively new journal, it had not yet been included in the major databases.

Research specific to the topic of culture and mentoring is not extensive, so we conducted multiple searches connecting a variety of words with mentoring. We excluded youth and students in the search process and limited the search to manuscripts in peer-reviewed journals published between 2000 and 2013 that were available in full text. We began the search using the terms *mentoring* and *culture* and *education*. We then conducted a series of searches replacing culture with *women, gender, diversity, race* and *ethnicity*, in turn. This yielded 415 manuscripts. After reading the abstracts, we eliminated those that did not deal with educational contexts. Since there were very few studies that focused specifically on cultural or contextual issues, we included several that dealt with the issue in a tangential way. Additionally, we examined articles that described programs in a variety of countries even if the manuscript was not research based, as they often provided important cultural understandings we found of value. At the end of this process, we selected 70 articles for further review.

Source: Kent, A. M., Kochan, F., and Green, A. M. (2013).

If you are looking for a quick and efficient way to search, obtain, and organize electronic sources, there are services specifically designed for this purpose. One such service is EndNote (*http://endnote.com*); however, it costs money to become a member. There are other services that are free. One example is Zotero (*www.zotero.org/about*), which describes itself as "a free and easy-to-use research tool that helps you collect, organize, and analyze research and lets you share it in a variety of ways." To back up articles or create your own bibliography, check out other choices such as cloud computing sources, Google Documents, and Dropbox. Evernotes is another example of a free document-saving cloud computing sources tool (*www.evernote.com*). According to the Evernotes website, the tool's "powerful search makes finding documents, text, and images lightning fast. Anytime, anywhere, and across all of your devices."

Another tool that you may find helpful is social bookmarking, an online catalog of hyperlinks that users want to share. Many social bookmarking applications allow individuals to vote on a link's usefulness or to comment on the accuracy of the information it conveys.

CREATING YOUR BIBLIOGRAPHY

There is a difference between the terms *bibliography* and *references*, although both are usually found at the end of the written work. Bibliography includes *all* the sources that you consulted and read during your study, even if you read them simply to gain background information. By comparison, references include only the works that were actually cited or referred to within the text (Ridley, 2012). Theses and dissertations, as well as grant proposals and scholarly articles, use references, rather than a bibliography.

The exact listing of each source at the end of your work will depend on the writing style that you use. Three of the main writing styles are those developed by the American Psychological Association (APA), the Modern Language Association (MLA), and the University of Chicago Press (*Chicago Manual of Style*). You can use available reference management systems that will allow you to create your bibliography in your chosen writing style. EndNote, mentioned above, lets you find literature on your topic, organize the sources, and build the bibliography in a style of your choice. You may also want to look at the Purdue University Online Writing Lab website (*https://owl.english.purdue.edu/owl*), which assists users in creating a bibliography in their selected style. This is a free website that is very helpful in using APA and MLA publication styles, as well as those in the *Chicago Manual of Style*. Another source is the Style Wizard (*www.stylewizard.com*), which is designed to help writers create a bibliography in APA or MLA styles. (See Chapter 11 for further information.) Consult with your professor, grant guidelines, or publication guidelines to determine which writing style you should use.

TO DO: *How to Record Literature Search Sources Electronically and Create Your Bibliography*

The checklist in Table 4.6 summarizes the steps in recording your search sources and creating your bibliography.

TABLE 4.6. Electronically Recording Your Literature Search Sources and Creating Your Bibliography	
Step	✓
1. Save and mail yourself the electronic documents that you find, when possible.	
2. Ask your local library to send you electronically articles that you wish to obtain but are not available as full text.	
3. Consider searching, obtaining, and organizing electronic sources using commercially available services.	
4. Create your bibliography as you obtain sources on your topic.	
5. Consult with your professor, grant guidelines, or publication guidelines to determine which bibliography style you should use (e.g., APA, MLA, or Chicago style).	
6. Consider using a reference management system that will allow you to create, organize, and build your bibliography in your chosen style.	

WHAT'S NEXT?

The focus of this chapter is on the library search process. We provided a detailed description of types of sources and offered techniques and strategies for finding sources in traditional and digital libraries and other online databases. In the next chapter we discuss the reading cycle, from selecting the sources to identifying relevant information in each source, to taking notes.

CHAPTER SUMMARY

1. There are several types of source materials, including books, articles, conference papers, reviews, and what is referred to as "gray literature." These sources are divided into primary, secondary, and tertiary sources.

2. Although digital search engines enable researchers to locate more information and to do so faster and more efficiently, the reliability, validity, and trustworthiness of the sources have to be established.

3. When searching for sources on your topic, it is a good idea to start with the most recent research you can find because it will include an updated literature review and references on your topic.

4. Throughout the process of your search, carefully record every source that you find to enable you to retrieve this information more easily later.

5. To search the fields in the records (e.g., titles, abstracts, and the author's name), use the most accurate *keywords* or search terms that relate to your research topic.

6. Another way to search a database is to use a *subject* or *descriptor,* which is a specific term used by the discipline or library catalog to categorize the source.

7. Another helpful source for locating keywords is a *thesaurus,* a dictionary containing a list of synonyms and related words.

8. You can search Google Scholar, Amazon, and Wikipedia as well as other, more general, online resources, such as those maintained by professional organizations and governments, which are widely available.

9. You can expand your search by using a truncated form of your keywords which is often done by adding an asterisk (*) to the truncated search word, or narrow your search by specifying the type of materials you want according to one or more categories.

10. Create a bibliography as you go along in your search process that includes all the sources you consulted and read during your study.

CHAPTER 5

Selecting, Analyzing, and Keeping Notes of Sources

By now you have identified sources on your topic through a library search and are ready to move to the next phase of the literature review process. This next phase entails immersing yourself in a purposeful, analytical, and critical reading of the sources you have found.

You may be a bit overwhelmed by the plethora of materials you have located, and the prospect of reviewing all of them may seem a grueling prospect. However, reading for a literature review is different from a regular reading of text since it is done for a specific goal, that of generating a product which is an analytical reading of the studies and theories on your chosen topic. As an efficient literature review writer, you should not read the literature for its own sake, but rather for a specific purpose and with a practical lens. This means extracting only relevant information from the selected sources in order to create your own original review of the literature (Blumberg, Cooper, & Schindler, 2008). While immersing yourself in the books, articles, and reports about your topic, ask yourself the following questions: What can I draw from the text that directly contributes to my own understanding of my research topic? What in the text may enable me to come closer to answering the research questions that guide my review (Jesson et al., 2011)?

The process of analyzing the literature on your topic requires several reading cycles, each with its own goals and purposes. Our discussion of the reading cycles is divided into two chapters: Chapter 5 outlines the steps involved in a purposeful and analytical reading of the literature, whereas Chapter 6 centers on the process of critical evaluation of the literature.

In this chapter we present the first reading cycle, which begins by scanning each individual source in order to determine whether to include it in the reading list. The next step is a quick reading of each of these chosen sources to identify the sections within them that are specifically relevant to your topic. These sections are then read carefully and notes are taken to analyze and summarize the information selected from each source. Thus, the narrative in this chapter is divided into four parts: (1) selection of sources, (2) identifying relevant information within individual sources, (3) note-taking, and (4) developing thematic concentric circles.

SELECTION OF SOURCES

You may be a bit intimidated by the number of printed or digital articles, research reports, and books that you have compiled, and the thought of selecting appropriate sources for review among "the exponentially growing body of literature" (Kwan, 2008, p. 42) may seem daunting. However, we hope that the guidance we provide in this chapter will make the task manageable. Here we explain the selection process by describing the steps involved in choosing the sources for your review. These steps are: (1) scanning the sources, (2) determining the scope of the review, and (3) using criteria for inclusion and exclusion.

Scanning the Sources

Once you obtain the references, start by scanning each individual source to determine its relevance and usefulness for your review. Check each source to determine whether it was peer reviewed or written by well-known researchers or theoreticians in the field. Once this is determined, skim each research article by reading the abstract, introduction, research question, and conclusions. You may also scan the article's headings and read a few sentences from each section. In considering the relevancy of a book, you may want to read the blurb on the back cover or book reviews. Additionally, you may go over the book's table of contents, skim the introduction, and perhaps the first or second paragraph of each chapter (Dawidowicz, 2010).

Remember, a text may be about the general topic of your research but still not useful to the discussion of the specific issues at the center of your review. Articles that are not related or are only slightly related to the topic of your study will cause your review to become less focused and ineffectively organized (Machi & McEvoy, 2012). At the same time, an article may be valuable for your review even if it does not explore exactly the same issues that are at the center of your research; it may provide some needed contextual information that contributes to a deeper understanding of your topic (Machi & McEvoy, 2012; Ridley, 2012). With each article you read, ask yourself: Does the information in this study correspond to the issue

I want to explore? Or alternatively, does it expand my knowledge and add some background information needed for a more comprehensive understanding of my topic?

Determining the Scope of the Review

Once you have established the credibility and usefulness of your references, you should decide on the level of coverage for your literature review. Cooper's (1988) taxonomy of literature reviews highlights four possible approaches to sources' level of coverage: (1) *exhaustive review*—reviewing all relevant sources; (2) *exhaustive with selective citation review*—setting the boundary of what references will be reviewed according to defined criteria; (3) *representative review*—choosing sources that are typical for particular groups of work in the literature; and (4) *central review*—focusing only on seminal works. The first two approaches are usually preferred by writers of systematic or meta-analysis reviews. Researchers writing traditional–narrative and hermeneutic–phenomenological reviews often choose representative or central reviews. Whichever approach you follow, we suggest that you explain thoughtfully and openly the rationale for your choice of level of coverage. (See Chapter 2 for a more comprehensive discussion of Cooper's taxonomy.)

Besides the type of literature review you intend to write, the purpose of the review may also dictate how thorough you should be. Are you preparing the literature review for your master's thesis or dissertation work? Is it part of a term paper or perhaps a required section of a grant proposal? Each of these types of reviews has a different purpose. Consulting with your professors or with the grant director may help you gain a clearer understanding of the required level of coverage.

Using Criteria for Inclusion or Exclusion

Determining what to include or exclude in the literature review is "probably the most distinct [aspect] of literature reviewing" (Boote & Beile, 2005, p. 7). When you skim through the references trying to decide which of them should be part of your literature review, it is a good idea to use consistent criteria for inclusion or exclusion of sources (Booth et al., 2008). Such criteria will enable you to have a transparent and thoughtful selection process.

In case you are writing a systematic review, your inclusion and exclusion criteria for selecting sources should be explicitly outlined and predetermined as your research questions are developed. These criteria may include items such as publication in peer-reviewed journals, target population, type of intervention or treatment, type of research design, outcome, and data synthesis (see the checklist in Table 5.1, p. 77). Choosing the studies to review, according to these criteria, will enhance your ability to answer your research questions and avoid wasting time on sources that are not likely to provide useful data.

TABLE 5.1. A Checklist for Assessing Whether a Source Should Be Included in a Systematic Review	
Inclusion and exclusion criteria	✓
Publication in a peer-reviewed journal	
Participants' age range	
Type of intervention/treatment	
Measurable and specified outcome (hypothesis)	
Type of research design	
Methods of data analysis	

With the other types of review, the criteria for inclusion and exclusion are more flexible but also more complex. Bruce (2001) proposes eight considerations for deciding whether a source should be included in your review. These considerations are centered on topicality, comprehensiveness, breadth, relevance, currency, exclusion, authority, and availability.

Topicality is concerned with the topic that is the focus of your review. You should check whether the article discusses the issues that are at the center of your research. For example, if you are exploring moral development of female teenagers, you may want to include topics such as Piaget's theory of moral development, Kohlberg's moral development stages, and Gilligan's feminist moral theory.

Comprehensiveness is concerned with the level of literature review coverage of your reading list. You may want to go over the four choices of levels of coverage outlined by Cooper (1988) and mentioned above (i.e., exhaustive review, exhaustive with selected citation review, representative review, and central review) and select the one that is most appropriate for your type of review. For example, if you plan to use qualitative research design for your study of moral development among female teenagers, a representative review will probably fit your needs. On the other hand, if you are leaning toward undertaking quantitative research, you may choose exhaustive review with selected citation review.

Breadth is concerned with useful information beyond the specific topic of your research. Such information may provide contextual background knowledge that supports the significance of your research topic. For example, if you are researching the issue of teacher mentoring, you may want to find out information about topics that are seemingly not directly related, such as attrition rate among new teachers and its implications for the school system.

Relevance is concerned with the relatedness of the sources to the focus of your research. Relevance is distinguished from "topicality" because the text you have designated as relevant may be drawing knowledge from research fields not directly related to your own discipline. For example, continuing with the topic of mentoring, you may decide that literature on stages of adult learning from the field of psychology may shed a valuable light on the topic of mentoring teachers.

Currency is concerned with the timeliness of the text used. While you may use classical texts and studies to highlight how your topic has evolved, you have to be sure that you include current, up-to-date research. For example, if your literature review is focused on gender occupational segregation, be sure to include studies published in the last 5 years.

Exclusion is concerned with explicit statements of what aspects are *not* included in the framework of your review and, consequently, what literature will be excluded. For example, in a review on women's occupational equality, you may state explicitly that your literature review will focus on studies conducted in the United States only and focused on occupational segregation based on gender only and not on other factors such as age, religion, or race. Additionally, you may indicate that you exclude studies that are not published in the English language.

Authority is concerned with seminal theorists, prominent researchers, or landmark studies that have shaped the development of your field of inquiry. When trying to understand the landscape of your topic, most researchers advise that you include studies or writings by central figures in your field. For example, if your study is about cultural anthropology, in your literature review you may want to refer to Margaret Mead and the research that was inspired by her work.

Availability is concerned with the ability to locate or obtain particular sources for your literature review. With the current technology and online resources this is less of a concern, but costs or time delays may still affect your choice to include a particular work in your reading list. For example, you may decide not to include a source on your topic because of difficulties of obtaining an out-of-print book or an unpublished paper.

All eight criteria for inclusion or exclusion are helpful when you choose the literature for your review. However, when you consider how these criteria may impact your own choice of sources, be aware that there is some tension between putting the emphasis on the comprehensiveness or on the relevancy of the sources you choose. Ravitch and Riggan (2017) note the debate that takes place among scholars over whether the emphasis in a literature review should be on a thorough synthesis of all literature related to one's topic as proposed by researchers such as Boote and Beile (2005) and Hart (1998) or on a selective review of sources that are most relevant to the research question as advocated by Maxwell (2006). Ravitch and Riggan assert, and we tend to agree, that the important question is not the number of sources that are included in the literature review, but rather how to arrive at an understanding of what is most relevant to the topic of the study and to the review writer's own research design.

As previously discussed (see Chapter 3), in a systematic review sharing the criteria and the rationale for inclusion or exclusion of sources is a requirement. While sharing such a rationale is not required of traditional–narrative and hermeneutic–phenomenological review writers, we suggest following Boote and Beile's (2005) recommendation that these writers do so. As you write your review, clearly outline its scope and demonstrate that the level of literature coverage and the criteria for inclusion and exclusion have been considered carefully and purposefully.

An example of an explanation of the scope of the review and the use of inclusion and exclusion criteria can be found in an article by Winkler-Wagner (2015) on the success of African American women in college (Box 5.1).

Table 5.2 (p. 80) outlines questions you may ask yourself when considering whether a reference should be included or excluded from your reading list.

Publication Bias

As you decide what sources to include, based on the eight criteria above, keep in mind the problem of publication bias, which is especially an issue in writing a systematic review. This problem refers to the fact that what gets published does not necessarily represent *all* the studies that were conducted on your topic. A phenomenon referred to as "the file-drawer problem" (Rosenthal, 1979) describes a situation where there are many studies that are never submitted for publication or never published. The reason is that investigators are less likely to submit their research if the results obtained are negative or not in the direction that was predicted, and reviewers and editors are not as likely to recommend or publish such studies. Therefore, the research that you may find in your literature search may be biased because it is not a random or representative sample of *all* the studies that were conducted on your topic (Song et al., 2009).

BOX 5.1. An Example of the Use of Inclusion and Exclusion Criteria

I developed criteria for inclusion and exclusion of studies in order to narrow the scope of the analysis. . . . Given the breadth of scholarship that has touched on various aspects of college access and success of undergraduates, I limited the scope of the review to literature pertaining to experiences and outcomes after college admission. To be included in the review, studies must have (a) explored or examined aspects of African American undergraduate women's experience after their enrollment in U.S. College; (b) been an empirical study, theoretical article, or historical analysis; (c) been published in a peer-reviewed journal or by an academic press; (d) been available for download from electronic database or library by March 2014; (e) examined phenomena pertaining specifically to educational success in college, such as achievement, self-concept, degree completion, or support structures; and (f) include discussion or analysis of college experiences with respect to race, gender, or both. I included articles from an array of academic disciplines in the review, provided that they met inclusion criteria. . . . I excluded from the review any literature that focused on issues of college access, college admission, or college choice, even when those studies sampled college students because these topics merit their own review.

Source: Winkler-Wagner (2015, p. 173).

TABLE 5.2. Questions to Consider When Determining Whether a Study Should Be Included in or Excluded from the Literature Review

Criteria	Question to ask
Topicality	Is the study concerned with the topic of my research?
Comprehensiveness	How does the study contribute to the thorough treatment of the topic at the center of my review?
Breadth	Does the study provide information relevant to understanding the general background of my research?
Relevance	Does the study present related information from other fields that is valuable to my topic?
Currency	Is the study current and up to date?
Exclusion	Is the study within the explicit framework of my research?
Authority	Is this a landmark study or was it written by or about a seminal theoretician or researcher in my field?
Availability	Is the source accessible?

Reaching a Saturation Point

Researchers, especially beginners, find it challenging to ascertain when they have read enough sources for their literature review. Their intellectual curiosity and love of knowledge inspire them to continuously look for more and more information. Ollhoff (2013) offers the concept of a *saturation point* as a clue for when it might be time to stop searching for more references. By saturation point Ollhoff means reaching the point when you keep reading the same ideas and you are no longer learning anything new about your topic. According to Garrard (2014), the only way of determining thoroughness is your own subjective sense of "knowing the literature well enough to own it" (p. 118).

GROUP WORK

1. Based on the eight criteria offered by Bruce (2001) and the example in Box 5.1, jot down a brief explanation of the rationale for the level of coverage you have chosen for your literature review and the inclusion and exclusion criteria you intend to follow.

2. Within your research group:
   a. Share your writing.
   b. Using two of the sources you have identified through the library search, explain how you have decided whether to include or exclude each of them in your reading list.

|||||||||||||||||||||||IDENTIFYING RELEVANT INFORMATION WITHIN INDIVIDUAL SOURCES

Once you have chosen a set of sources that you have deemed pertinent for your review, immerse yourself in reading and analyzing the selected texts. This process is ongoing throughout the literature review process.

Next, we discuss ways to identify and take notes of relevant information from individual sources that you have selected. We begin with suggestions of a systematic method of organizing those references into folders.

Creating a Document Folder

Before starting with the reading, you may want to create a document folder that will comprise all electronic sources such as articles, e-book chapters, full-text dissertations, and government reports that you have decided are worth reading and reviewing (Garrard, 2014). You may also create a traditional nonelectronic folder for those documents that are not available electronically, such as hard copies of book chapters or paper presentations. Arrange the documents alphabetically by the author's last name within both electronic and nonelectronic folders (Ridley, 2012).

According to Garrard, the main advantage of keeping document folders is the ability to easily locate texts whenever needed throughout the literature review process. The document folder also helps in managing the process of summarizing, analyzing, and synthesizing the texts in an efficient way. Furthermore, using document folders makes it easy to insert additional materials as you continue reading and identifying other appropriate references.

There are several effective reference management software systems. Among them are:

▶ EndNote: *www.endnote.com*
▶ Evernote: *https://evernote.com/evernote*
▶ Reference Manager: *www.refman.com*
▶ RefWorks: *www.refworks.com*
▶ Zotero: *www.zotero.org/about*

Such systems would be very helpful for developing your electronic documents folder and make the next step of identifying relevant information within individual sources and note-taking easier to carry out.

Reading and Rereading the Texts

Once you have taken care of storing and organizing the selected literature material and created a document folder, you are now ready to immerse yourself in reading and rereading each text. The common process recommended by most researchers consists of the following steps: First, quickly read the entire document to familiarize yourself with its overall content. Then, reread the text to identify sections that are useful and relevant for your own review. You may allow these identified sections to emerge through your reading or you may use predetermined key terms drawn from the research questions that guide your review. Examine each source with questions related to the methodology or content, such as the following, which are based on recommendations suggested by Jesson et al. (2011).

1. What *issues* in this document may contribute to my review?
2. Are there *definitions* of concepts that are at the center of my review?
3. What *information* may contribute to the background knowledge needed for my research?
4. Are there *historical* factors that may be applicable to my review?
5. What *theories* or *philosophical* assertions described in the text are relevant to my review?
6. What *methods* were used in the study that are of interest for my own research?
7. Are the *findings* relevant to my research question(s)?
8. Are there facts or statistical information that may contribute to highlighting the *significance* of my topic?

Once you have identified the sections that are valuable for your review of the literature, mark them clearly. When using your own paper copies or electronic texts, use colored highlights, different-colored fonts, or shades to indicate the paragraphs that you deem relevant. In case of loaned material that needs to be returned, you may use stickers in different shapes or colors that will help you locate the sections you selected.

Now go back and reread deeply and carefully the identified passages to ensure their usefulness to your review. Jot down in the margin of the page (or the colored stickers) key terms or categories that capture the essence of the passage.

GROUP WORK

1. Share with your group two to three articles you chose for your review and explain:
    a. What information in these articles contributes to a better understanding of your topic? Share paragraphs that illustrate these contributions.
    b. What information within these paragraphs is relevant to the methodology or content of your research?
2. Share with the group your plans for organizing your document folders.

NOTE-TAKING

After reading the articles, selecting and demarking the appropriate sections, and identifying them by key terms or categories, you are ready for note-taking. As you take notes, remember that your focus is not the article itself but rather the sections you have identified as relevant to your topic. In your notes, interpret and summarize the relevant issues as presented by the source's authors and reflect on their meaning for your literature review.

Taking notes may seem a laborious and time-consuming process but, in fact, these notes form a valuable basis for your review writing. Compiling these notes will enhance your ability to:

▶ Make connections across sources and identify similarities and differences among them.

▶ Arrange the information around themes and subthemes.

▶ Develop a logical organization for your review.

▶ Reference the sources and avoid unintentional plagiarism.

▶ Easily locate information at a later date.

▶ Present the information in a coherent and organized manner.

The Process of Note-Taking

For each article you have selected, you should take notes as soon as you finish reading and rereading it, while the text is still fresh in your mind. In your note-taking, do not summarize the article but rather focus on the information in the text that you have identified as relevant. You do not need to read the full article again, but rather concentrate on those sections that you have previously highlighted. Extract salient information from these highlighted sections and disregard the rest.

The information you want to extract from the literature is probably spread across many sources and consists of myriad details. In order to write effective notes you need to stay organized and impose order on this plethora of information. To enhance this organization process, we suggest using article note-taking index cards (ANTICs). These ANTICs offer a systematic and consistent format that will ensure that the information is orderly structured.

While we recognize that there are those who still prefer writing their notes by hand, we strongly recommend taking advantage of the efficiency that electronic index cards offer. They make recording, sorting, locating, rearranging, and retrieving information quicker and more effective. The ANTIC template (see Figure 5.1, p. 85) for both handwritten and electronic index cards is similar, and the process of constructing it is discussed next.

1. Prepare a separate index card for each individual article and number it.

2. The top section includes information about the source (author, year of publication, title) and the research question or purpose of the study.

3. Divide the space under this section into three columns: (a) in the left column, identify the key term of each issue; (b) in the central column, write a summary of the text related to this particular issue, including chosen quotations; (c) in the right-hand column write your reflections on the ideas presented.

4. The number of rows in each table corresponds to the number of issues in this source that you deemed relevant for your review. Identify and label each issue.

5. An additional row is left empty at the bottom of the template in which you will write your assessment of the source. (The issue of assessing the articles is discussed at length in Chapter 6.)

The length of each ANTIC will vary from article to article, depending on the number of issues you have identified as relevant and their importance for your research. A detailed description of the content of each column is discussed next. We start by explaining the central column titled Analysis and Summary; next we clarify how Key Terms are determined; and we end with highlighting the role of the Reflection in the analysis process.

Analysis and Summary

Interpret and summarize each issue that you identified as relevant in the article. Be selective and highlight only the ideas and facts that are pertinent for understanding your topic. Be sure that the notes are clearly written so you will be able to easily recall the gist of your notes even when revisiting them after a long time. (You may

Author(s) _____		
Year of publication _____		
Title of the article/chapter _____		
Research question _____		

Key terms and categories	Analysis and summary	Reflection/response
Issue I:	 _____ Quotation (+ page number):	
Issue II:	 _____ Quotation (+ page number):	
Issue III:	 _____ Quotation (+ page number):	
Article assessment		

FIGURE 5.1. Template for article note-taking index cards (ANTICs).

want to note the page numbers in case you want to go back to the original source to reread the text.) Additionally, while at this point you should not worry about the actual writing of the review; effective notes may, in fact, become incorporated into the review narrative (Ollhoff, 2013).

The notes from each article may focus on methodological issues, such as theory of knowledge (epistemology), research design, data collection methods, findings, limitations, or implications. For quantitative studies, you may want to note whether the study was experimental or descriptive, the validity and reliability of the instruments, the sample used to gather data, or the statistical results and their significance. When it comes to qualitative studies, you may want to note the subjectivity of the researchers and the methods of establishing the trustworthiness of the study. Unique to the analysis of qualitative and hermeneutical–phenomenological studies is the emphasis on the social and theoretical contexts and the cultural constructions which should be noted. Additionally, record key metaphors, phrases, perspectives, inferred concepts, and core meanings that later will allow you to juxtapose, compare, and contrast between studies (Booth et al., 2016; Noblit & Hare, 1988; Walsh & Downe, 2005).

When taking notes on theoretical or conceptual issues, you may focus on definitions of terms that are at the heart of your study. These terms can be defined differently by various researchers and, consequently, highlight diverse perspectives on the same topic. Another issue you may note in the ANTIC is the social, political, or cultural context of the topic of your study or its evolution over time. At times, you may record the philosophical lens that frames the discussion in the articles, whereas for other references you may choose to focus on issues of policy and their implications for your research.

Table 5.3 (p. 87), based on suggestions by Jesson et al. (2011) and Booth et al. (2016), presents aspects that can assist you in identifying specific methodological and content issues that are relevant in each source.

Your interpretation of the author's writing should be articulated in your own words. The length of the summary—whether concise or more expansive—depends on its importance for your own study. Ridley (1912) suggests that when you take notes of relevant information within each article, your narrative should represent three degrees of depth and detail: *long-shot* references, *medium-shot* references, and *close-shot* references. In the case of *long-shot* references, the source is reviewed in general terms, acknowledging that the study took place without going into specific details. *Medium-shot* references are more relevant to your focus, and therefore more information about the research article is offered and the impact of the study on your research is considered. *Close-shot* references have particular bearing on your literature review, and, consequently, your discussion should include a detailed and critical examination and in-depth analysis of the reference.

TABLE 5.3. Identifying Methodological and Content Issues in Sources	
Methodology	**Content**
■ Theories of knowledge (epistemology)	■ Definition
■ Study design	■ Historical development
■ Reliability and validity	■ Theory
■ Location of study	■ Concept
■ Participants	■ Philosophical perspective
■ Data collection strategies	■ Social and cultural contexts
■ Data analysis procedures	■ Argument
■ Researcher's subjectivity	■ Standpoint
■ Trustworthiness	■ Policy
■ Metaphors, phrases, perspectives, and meanings	
■ Findings	
■ Limitations	
■ Implications	

Quotation

Occasionally, you may encounter a unique phrase or sentence that beautifully illustrates the author's idea. You may quote it in your narrative, but be sure that your quotation is precise and that the page number is noted, when available. (See Chapter 11 for further information about recording quotations.)

Key Terms

After summarizing and interpreting the selected sections in each article, categorize your notes and label them with key terms that will be recorded in the left-hand column of the ANTIC. The labels should reflect the content of the categorized sections and capture their essence. You may use predetermined key terms or allow them to emerge from the text. After you take notes on several articles, you will, most likely, identify repeating key terms and issues. Be sure that you use the same terms consistently.

This process of categorizing and labeling will help you later when you structure the organization of the literature review around themes and subthemes. It will also allow you to search the electronic indexes using keywords to develop various logical combinations from the summaries of all or part of the individual summaries you have written (Hart, 1998).

Reflection

In the right-hand column of the ANTIC, insert your own thoughts and insights about what you have summarized. Here you may also reflect on how the particular issue that you analyzed links to other articles you have read and note agreements, disagreements, and contrasting and complementary aspects. Your assessment of the articles will be done based on criteria discussed in Chapter 6. Record the article evaluations at the bottom of the ANTIC.

Table 5.4 (p. 89) is an example of an ANTIC used by a literature review writer taking notes on sections of an article on the topic of mentoring.

GROUP WORK

1. Present to your group the ANTICs you have constructed for at least two of the articles included in your review. Share the following:
   a. The summaries of relevant sections, the quotations you have chosen, and your reasons for choosing them.
   b. The labels you have given to the key terms and the issues you summarized in this article.
   c. The contribution of this information to your literature review.
   d. A comparison of the information gained from this article to what was learned from other sources regarding the same issues.
2. Discuss with the group whether there are other points that you should be looking for in the literature.

Digital Note-Taking

Nowadays there are dozens of options for creating your own system of note-taking using digital notebooks or software packages. These electronic programs can help you locate quickly and efficiently the key terms and issues you have identified and the information you summarized in the ANTICs. These electronic programs include Evernotes, Google Docs, OneNote, Simplenote, Workflow, and Zotero. Following is a brief explanation of each.

▶ **Evernotes** (*www.evernote.com*) is a flexible and effortless note-taking and syncing tool. The note-taking feature enables users to type in notes and scan in handwritten text. In addition to its web app, the program has apps for Windows Mac, iOS, Android, and Windows phones.

▶ **Google Docs** (*https://docs.google.com/forms*) is a free and easy-to-use tool for note-taking that can be used to create and edit documents online and then organize the documents according to themes.

Key terms and categories	Reference	Analysis and summary	Reflection/response
TABLE 5.4. An Example of Note-Taking Using ANTIC			
Theme 1: Definition of mentorship	Ambrosetti, A., & Dekkers, J. (2010). The interconnectness of the role of mentors and mentees in pre-service teacher education. *Australian Journal of Teacher Education, 35*(6), 42–55	The definition of mentoring is interconnected to the contextual factors that influence mentoring in teacher education. However, although there are numerous definitions, they do not clearly outline the actions that occur during the mentoring process. The authors' definition highlights the hierarchical and reciprocal relationships between the mentor and the mentee, who work together toward a defined outcome for the mentorship. Some other definitions of mentoring are: Mentoring is a process (Smith, 2007). Mentoring is a process but also a relationship (Kwan & Lopez-Real, 2005). Mentoring is contextual (Fairbank et al., 2000). Mentoring is relational, developmental, and contextual (Lai, 2005). **Quotation** (p. 52): "The relationship usually follows a developmental pattern within a specific timeframe and roles as defined, expectations are outlined and purpose is ideally clearly delineated."	Need to find the etymological source of the word "mentor" and its implication for current definitions. I like the assertion that the definition is part of the contextual factors. Need to expand this idea in my literature review chapter. I need to read the original articles that were noted in my summary.
Theme 2: Mentor roles	Ambrosetti, A., & Dekkers, J. (2010). The interconnectedness of the role of mentors and mentees in pre-service teacher education, *Australian Journal of Teacher Education, 35*(6), 42–55.	Based on multiple articles, the authors present a list of common perceptions of the mentor role: **Supporter:** Assist the mentee to grow personally and professionally. **Role model:** Assist by example and demonstration of desired behavior. **Facilitator:** Provides opportunities to mentees to grow by performing their tasks. **Assessor:** Assesses the mentee's performance and offers critique. **Collaborator:** Shares and reflects with the mentee in a collaborative relationship. **Friend:** Behaves as a critical friend. **Trainer:** Provides skills and resources. **Protector:** Protects the mentee from unpleasant situations. **Colleague:** Treats the mentee as an equal professional.	Interesting list. May be helpful in categorizing the mentors observed. Will I be able to group under the three perspectives suggested by Brondyk, S., & Searby, L. (2013)?
Article assessment			

▶ **OneNote** (*http://office.microsoft.com/en-us/onenote*) is free and available for Microsoft Office users, allowing them to customize and organize their note-taking according to their need. It enables you to store text, pictures, and audio and video recordings.

▶ **Simplenote** (*https://simplenote.com*) is free and it allows users to back up and share notes for reading or editing and to sync data automatically across devices.

▶ **Workflow** (*www.workflowgen.com*) is a part of Word that offers a variety of ways to organize data by using different ways of searching keywords and information from the data you have entered.

▶ **Zotero** (*www.zotero.org/about*) is part of Firefox web browser that enables you to extract and manage Internet and online sources, save references, and take notes on documents.

THEMATIC CONCENTRIC CIRCLES

In addition to analyzing individual sources and constructing an ANTIC for each reference, you may also want to consider what might be the major themes around which your literature review will evolve. The use of ANTICs allows for key terms, categories, and then themes to emerge. However, during the process of analysis, there is also an advantage in tentatively identifying major themes that will serve as the foundations of your review. These major themes are just beginning to emerge at this point and may be changed, rephrased, or even eliminated as you continue reading and analyzing your references and become more knowledgeable about your topic. Still, identifying the central themes will give you a sense of the whole while you explore its individual components. The strategy of using *concentric circles* may help you formulate the overarching foci you want to cover in your literature review.

Concentric circles comprise a series of circles, one inside the other, with a common center point. The innermost circle, the center point, contains the central topic or your research question, while the surrounding circles present the major themes that are drawn from that focus (see Figure 5.2, p. 91). The steps involved in creating the concentric circles are described in Table 5.5.

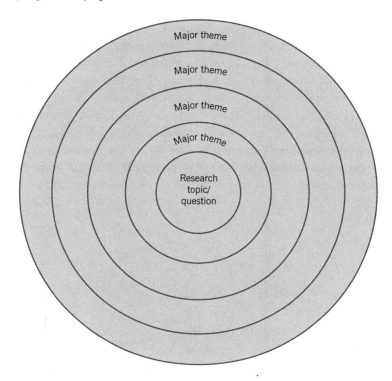

FIGURE 5.2. Thematic concentric circles.

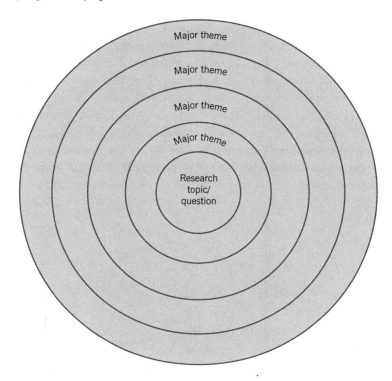 TO DO: *Forming Thematic Concentric Circles*

Table 5.5 presents the steps in forming your thematic concentric circles.

TABLE 5.5. Steps Involved in Forming Thematic Concentric Circles	
Step	✓
1. Start by drawing a small circle and write in it your research questions or the study's focused topic.	
2. Around this inner circle, draw four to seven concentric circles that fit inside each other.	
3. Choose what themes need to be explored in order to gain a deeper understanding of your research topic or question. Ask yourself: "What do I and my readers need to know about my topic" and "What do I want them to understand in order to create the scholarly context that leads to my own study?"	
4. In each concentric circle, write one of the themes you identified. Keep in mind that at this point there is no need to consider the hierarchy among the themes. (The issue of the order of the themes is discussed in Chapter 7, which focuses on the organization and structure of the literature review.)	

An example of thematic concentric circles was created by Michelle, a high
school teacher and a doctoral student in a curriculum studies program. She decided
to focus her dissertation on the use of young adult literature to encourage social
discourse among the students. She decided to utilize thematic concentric circles to
identify the major issues around which she would write her literature review. In
the innermost circle, she wrote "Adolescent lit for dialogical discourse," which is
the topic of her dissertation research. Around it, she drew five circles and within
them she wrote the emerging major themes of her literature review. She drew those
themes from the readings and the ANTICs she had done so far and what she intui-
tively felt was essential for understanding her topic (see Figure 5.3).

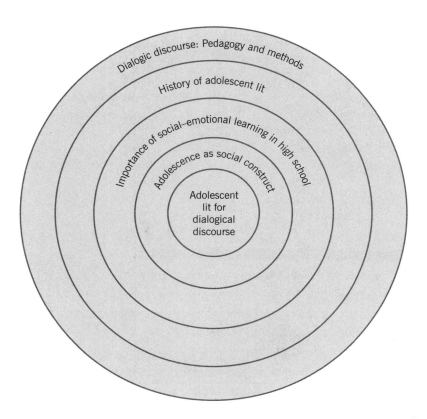

FIGURE 5.3. An example of thematic concentric circles.

WHAT'S NEXT?

This chapter describes the first reading cycle and provides strategies for selecting, organizing, and analyzing your sources. Literature review, though, is not merely an analytical summary of what you have read; rather, it should aim to critically assess the research you are reviewing, identify strengths, and reveal weaknesses. Critical review of the sources is the focus of our next chapter.

CHAPTER SUMMARY

1. The process of analyzing the literature on your topic requires several reading cycles, each with its own goal and purpose.

2. The steps involved in choosing the sources for your review are (a) scanning the sources, (b) determining the scope of the review, and (c) using criteria for inclusion and exclusion.

3. According to Cooper's taxonomy (1988), there are four possible approaches to the level of a literature review's coverage: (a) *exhaustive review*—reviewing all relevant sources; (b) *exhaustive with selective citation review*—setting the boundary of what references will be reviewed according to defined criteria; (c) *representative review*—choosing sources that are typical; and (d) *central review*—focusing only on seminal works.

4. In a systematic review, the inclusion and exclusion criteria should be explicitly outlined and predetermined as research questions are developed.

5. Eight considerations for inclusion and exclusion are applied to other types of reviews, centering on topicality, comprehensiveness, breadth, relevance, currency, exclusion, authority, and availability.

6. Create an electronic document folder that will include all of your electronic sources and a nonelectronic folder for documents that are not available electronically; both folders should be organized alphabetically by the authors' last names.

7. Immerse yourself in reading and rereading your sources to identify and mark relevant sections and examine each with questions related to its methodology and content.

8. The process of finding sources is iterative and may continue throughout the development of the literature review.

9. Taking notes of each article forms a valuable basis for your review writing and should start as soon as you finish reading the text, and you may find the article note-taking index card (ANTIC) useful for effective notes writing, staying organized, and imposing order on the information gathered.

10. Consider using thematic concentric circles for identifying tentatively major themes of your literature review.

CHAPTER 6

Evaluating Research Articles

Once you have extracted, summarized, and analyzed relevant information from the sources that you deemed valuable for your study, you are now ready to critically evaluate the literature. Reading for the purpose of extracting and summarizing the relevant information demands paying attention to the details of the study, while reading for critical assessment comprises a "holistic judgment of the study" (Booth et al., 2016, p. 129). On the other hand, some literature review writers prefer to critically assess the quality of the studies they review at the same time they summarize them because, from their perspective, doing these two processes concurrently is more efficient and saves time (Booth et al., 2016).

In this book we have chosen to divide our discussion into two chapters: In Chapter 5, we discussed the procedures involved in extraction, analysis, and summarization of the sources; and in this chapter, we turn our focus to the critical reading of texts. We believe that doing so increases the level of clarity and understanding of the process involved in each step. You, on the other hand, should feel free to choose whether you want to combine the steps or work on each separately.

In any way you choose to proceed, be aware that the purpose of a review is to provide a critique, rather than a mere report, on the literature on your topic (Wellington, Bathmaker, Hunt, McCulloch, & Sikes, 2005). Critiquing the research sources means gauging the quality of the references and the soundness of the findings reported. In this chapter we first highlight the role of a critical evaluation of the literature on your topic. We then outline criteria that may help you in evaluating quantitative, qualitative, and mixed-methods research, and in examining the validity of these studies. Then we analyze the unique ways of assessing hermeneutic–phenomenological research.

|||||||||||||||||||||||||||||||||||||||||||||||||CRITICAL EVALUATION OF THE QUALITY OF SOURCES

When you write a literature review it is important that you adopt a critical stance toward the sources you review (Ridley, 2012). This means having confidence in your own ability to make a deliberate and informed judgment while at the same time keeping a degree of humility and respect toward researchers whose work you are critiquing (Wellington et al., 2005).

You should assess the strengths and flaws of each individual study in order to evaluate its claims, assess its methodology, and ascertain the validity and credibility of the findings. The quality and integrity of your review depends, to a large extent, on the sources you use. The claims you put forth in your writing draw their trustworthiness from the data you present as evidence (Booth et al., 2008; Machi & McEvoy, 2012). You should ensure that poorly designed research with unreliable evidences will not negatively impact the quality of your review or lead to misleading arguments (Galvan & Galvan, 2017).

At the same time, while you should be a critical reviewer, you should not be a hypercritical one (Booth et al., 2008). Your role as a literature review writer is not to look for perfect studies (Petticrew & Roberts, 2006) or to highlight every flaw in each research article that you review. Almost all studies have some weaknesses and your role is to consider which flaws are crucial and which have a minimal effect on the findings (Booth et al., 2016). While some researchers (e.g., Cooper, 1988) suggest eliminating studies with severe methodological inadequacies from the literature review, others (e.g., Booth et al., 2016; Hart, 1998; McMillan & Wergin, 2010) assert that even when the study has imitations, it can still provide valuable information. In fact, Walsh and Downe (2005), when discussing the appraisal of qualitative research, recommend that even if there are serious flaws in studies, they may still be worth including in the review in order to highlight the need for better-quality studies in the future.

In short, what is important is the impact of the findings from each article upon your own review's claims, arguments, and conclusions. As you write your review, acknowledge the weaknesses, as well as the strengths, of these studies and demonstrate their relative impact on your work. This explicit awareness of the quality of the reviewed studies becomes what Dawidowicz (2010, p. 90) refers to as the "logical bridge" that allows your readers to understand how you have drawn your arguments from your sources and reached trustworthy conclusions.

While you may want to assess the quality of *all* the sources that are part of your literature review, we suggest that the detailed evaluation of articles be done mostly for those studies that are critical for your own review and have a central role in planning your future research. Additionally, we agree with Galvan and Galvan's (2017) recommendation that rather than critique each article on its own, it might, at times, be better to critique groups of sources together, especially when you identify a pattern of weakness that is common across these studies.

Furthermore, as you review individual articles, be cognizant of the style of your literature review. For example, systematic literature reviewers are basing their appraisal on precise and strict standards of evaluation (Jesson et al., 2011). By comparison, hermeneutic–phenomenological reviewers, while recognizing the importance of using rigorous sources, emphasize the idea that all articles may be included in the review (Walsh & Downe, 2005). Writers of traditional–narrative reviews assume a flexible stance and use different criteria for evaluating the quality of quantitative, qualitative, and mixed methods.

In this chapter, recognizing that each research type has its own quality standards, we follow the traditional–narrative reviewers and suggest criteria for appraising studies on the basis of their approach to research. We also offer guidelines for evaluating hermeneutic–phenomenological writings.

Most researchers (e.g., Booth et al., 2008; Cooper, 1984) contend that the quality of the design and methodology of the study and the validity and trustworthiness of the findings should be the primary criteria for judging its adequacy and the level of trust in its results. Therefore, in their discussion of literature critique, their focus is on ways to assess the study's design and methodology. While we agree with this assertion, we chose to follow McMillan and Wergin (2010) and in this chapter we provide criteria for assessing every section of research articles. We do so because we believe it is important to examine all the elements of research studies to determine their quality, and that this knowledge is essential for literature reviewers. We also believe that knowing the criteria for assessing all the elements of a study will help you assess your own work and improve the quality of your study.

CRITERIA FOR EVALUATING INDIVIDUAL STUDIES ||||||||||||||||||||||||||||||||||||||||||||||||||||||||||

In the following sections we provide criteria for assessing the quality of articles that can be categorized as quantitative, qualitative, mixed-methods, and hermeneutic–phenomenological studies. You may recall that Chapter 2 highlights the differences among quantitative, qualitative, and mixed-methods research. As we pointed out, each type of research is distinguished in its nature and purpose and those distinctions impact the way the research is conducted. All of these types of research include some form of quality standards; those standards are drawn out of the traditions, orientations, expectations, and norms that typify each approach to research (McMillan & Wergin, 2010). As we evaluate the different types of studies, these differences should be considered.

In quantitative research, demonstrating the quality of studies is an essential part of the research process and the criteria for assessing the studies are well established. On the other hand, there is considerable debate among qualitative researchers as to whether and how qualitative research should be evaluated (e.g., Booth et al., 2016; Denzin, 2009; Marshall & Rossman, 2015; McMillan & Schumacher, 2010).

From the qualitative researcher's point of view, truth is multiple and knowledge is socially constructed (Walsh & Downe, 2005). This assumption results in three basic positions on the value of assessment. The first camp (e.g., Dixon-Woods, Shaw, Agarwal, & Smith, 2004; Dixon-Woods, Bonas, et al., 2006; Teddlie & Tashakkori, 2009) contends that, in essence, *research is research,* and the set of shared criteria used by quantitative researchers (i.e., internal and external validity, credibility, transferability, conformability, and transparency) should be applied equally to qualitative studies.

The second camp asserts that there is an essential difference in the nature and purpose of qualitative and quantitative research. Therefore, a different set of criteria, unique to qualitative research, should be used to assess the soundness and trustworthiness of this type of study (e.g., Bazeley, 2013; Creswell, 2018; Lincoln & Guba, 1985; Marshall & Rossman, 2015; Maxwell, 2013).

The third camp of qualitative researchers believes that applying an explicit set of criteria to qualitative research is incompatible with the nature and purpose of this type of inquiry. They reject any kind of regulatory expectations implied by using assessment criteria (e.g., Denzin, 2009; Hammersley, 2007).

In this book we accept the notion that qualitative research should meet criteria for good research practice. With that in mind, and following Lincoln and Guba (1985), we believe that qualitative studies should not be judged using traditional standards borrowed from quantitative approaches. Rather, assessment of qualitative studies should be done using an alternative set of criteria reflecting the fact that qualitative methods are inherently subjective and local in scope; and validity and reliability should be defined within this framework.

Our discussion of evaluative criteria is divided into three parts. First, we provide criteria for those sections of the articles that are common to quantitative, qualitative, mixed-methods, and hermeneutic–phenomenological research, while also pointing out particular aspects that may differ among these types. Secondly, we provide separate criteria for evaluating the methodology and findings sections that differentiate quantitative, qualitative, and mixed-methods research. We also include a section about assessing the validity of these types of research. Thirdly, we present a short discussion that highlights criteria for assessing hermeneutic–phenomenological research. Each section concludes with a checklist that is designed to summarize the different processes of quality assessment for that specific type of research.

ELEMENTS OF RESEARCH ARTICLES COMMON TO QUANTITATIVE, QUALITATIVE, MIXED-METHODS, AND HERMENEUTIC–PHENOMENOLOGICAL RESEARCH ||||||||||||||||

There are certain elements that are expected to be included in most types of research articles, and the criteria used to assess them are therefore similar. On the other hand, there are parts that are unique to articles from different traditions of research, and the assessment criteria are therefore different. Following, we present the criteria to assess the elements that are common to quantitative, qualitative, mixed-methods, and hermeneutic–phenomenological research, while at the same time we point out the differences that distinguish each.

Title

The title is the reader's first introduction to the content of the article and thus should represent it accurately; it should be informative and fully explanatory. Most readers are likely to encounter the title for the first time when they conduct an electronic search on their topic, and a misleading title can cause the writer to overlook valuable articles or to invest unnecessary time and energy in obtaining references that are not relevant. Titles should be concise and avoid words that do not serve a useful purpose such as "A Study of . . ." It is recommended that the title not include more than 12 words (*Publication Manual of the American Psychological Association* [APA], 2010, p. 23). When possible, use complete rather than abbreviated terms. The use of colons in the title allows for conciseness as well as explanations.

Abstract

An abstract provides a preview and a summary of the study. The length of the abstract is commonly restricted by the journal where it is published, ranging most often from 50 to 150 words. Abstracts should accurately summarize the article and contain information about the purpose of the study, a brief description of the study's methodology, and the main findings (McMillan & Schumacher, 2010). A good abstract should be accurate, nonevaluative, coherent, readable, and concise (American Psychological Association, 2010, p. 26).

Introduction

The introduction provides a general context for the study, including a review of past literature and a definition of key terms and concepts. The introduction also includes a problem statement that defines the purpose of the study, the rationale for conducting it, and its significance for the researcher and for the field. This statement should also communicate the study's design (e.g., experimental or inter-pretive) and the variables to be studied (McMillan & Wergin, 2010).

Although in dissertations, theses, and grant proposals the introduction is a separate chapter, in published research articles the introduction and literature review are often combined into a single section. The research questions and—where appropriate—hypotheses may be included in this section or they may follow the literature review.

Literature Review

A well-structured literature review provides the background information about the topic of the study, placing it in the broader scholarly literature. A good review includes a critical analysis of previous studies (McMillan & Wergin, 2010), notes gaps in knowledge, inconsistencies, or the need to confirm previous findings, and builds a case for conducting the proposed study. A literature review typically starts with more general information about the topic and ends with a focused discussion of studies that are most related to the planned research.

Research Questions and Hypotheses

While the general purpose of the study may be stated in the introduction, the study's specific research questions and/or hypotheses are usually found after the literature review and are based on the information presented there. Although hypotheses are appropriate in most empirical quantitative studies, other nonexperimental studies may contain research questions but not hypotheses (McMillan & Schumacher, 2010). In studies where hypotheses are stated, they should be phrased in a way that allows them to be tested.

Research questions in qualitative, as well as in hermeneutic–phenomenological research, are mostly open-ended. It is common to start the research with questions of *what* and *how* and avoid phrasing them in a way that leads to yes or no answers. While the questions serve as a boundary around the inquiry, they should be general enough to allow flexibility in the research process (Efron & Ravid, 2013; Marshall & Rossman, 2011). It is common for questions in qualitative and hermeneutic–phenomenological research to evolve and change throughout the research process (Boell & Cecez-Kecmanovic, 2010, 2014).

In mixed-methods studies, there are likely to be two or more research ques-tions, each calling for a different approach to data collection (Efron & Ravid, 2013). A use of mixed methods allows researchers to pose both specific and open-ended questions. The questions can be determined at the start of the study or emerge once the study is under way (Creswell & Plano Clark, 2011).

TO DO: *Evaluating Common Elements in Quantitative, Qualitative, Mixed-Methods, and Hermeneutic–Phenomenological Research*

Table 6.1 provides a checklist for evaluating elements that are common to quantitative, qualitative, mixed-methods, and hermeneutic–phenomenological research.

TABLE 6.1. A Checklist for Evaluating Common Elements in Research Articles Reporting on Quantitative, Qualitative, Mixed-Methods, and Hermeneutic–Phenomenological Research

	Common article elements	✓
Title	▪ Is concise, clear, and accurately summarizes the main idea of the article	
Abstract	▪ Summarizes the article accurately and concisely within the prescribed number of words	
	▪ Is nonevaluative	
	▪ Includes information about the study's purpose	
	▪ Includes information about the study's methodology	
	▪ Includes information about the study's major findings	
Introduction	▪ The rationale for the study is presented, including its importance and relevance	
	▪ Key terms and concepts are explained	
	▪ The problem to be studied is stated and its significance is examined	
Literature review	▪ The research topic is placed in a broad scholarly context	
	▪ Provides comprehensive background information to evaluate the current research	
	▪ Important previous research findings are noted	
	▪ Critically discusses and evaluates related research studies	
	▪ Well organized in a logical order	
	▪ Includes up-to-date studies	
Research questions and/ or hypotheses (may be included in the introduction or follow the literature review)	▪ The research questions are clearly stated	
	▪ In quantitative research, the hypotheses are related to the research questions and are testable	
	▪ In qualitative and hermeneutic–phenomenological research, the questions are open-ended, often starting with *what* and *how*	
	▪ In qualitative and hermeneutic–phenomenological research the questions evolve and change throughout the research process	
	▪ Research questions are both open-ended and specific in mixed-methods approach	
	▪ There may be more than one research question in mixed-methods research, each calling for a different approach to data collection	

SECTIONS OF RESEARCH ARTICLES THAT CHARACTERIZE QUANTITATIVE, QUALITATIVE, AND MIXED-METHODS RESEARCH

Quantitative Research: Methodology, Results, Discussion, Validity, and Reliability

Methodology

This section describes how the study was conducted and includes information about the study's participants, data collection tools, data collection procedures, and data analysis. The description should be specific and detailed to allow other researchers to duplicate the study without having to contact the authors of the article (Garrard, 2014). It is important to note whether the study was experimental or nonexperimental. Experimental studies allow researchers to test cause-and-effect relationships between variables, whereas descriptive or nonexperimental studies are used to describe phenomena and test noncausal relationships between variables. While experimental methods are the best choice for studying cause-and-effect relationships, it is sometimes impossible or not practical to use such designs (Galvan, 2014) and nonexperimental methods have to be implemented.

Next we provide information about each subsection of the methodology: participants, data collection tools, data collection procedures, and data analysis. A brief discussion of the ethics of conducting quantitative research is also included.

PARTICIPANTS

It is important to provide specific information about the participants to allow for the generalization of the findings and replication of the study (American Psychological Association, 2010). This subsection should report on the demographic characteristics of the sample, the number of participants, and how they were selected. The reason for doing this is that results from a small sample are not considered as strong as those from a large sample. In another example, using volunteers in a study may introduce a degree of bias. Additionally, information about the participants may be study specific. For example, the age or gender of the participants may be important characteristics in one study but not in another.

DATA COLLECTION TOOLS

A variety of instruments may be used to collect data in quantitative studies, including surveys, tests, ratings, and archival materials (McMillan & Wergin, 2010). Structured interviews and observations may also yield quantitative data. A detailed description of the tool(s) used to collect data should be provided along with sample items.

Most data collection tools used by researchers fall into three general categories: (1) existing instruments that were developed by others, (2) modified existing instruments, and (3) new tools developed specifically for the study (Creswell & Plano Clark, 2011).

Using Existing Instruments. This approach allows the researchers to skip the step of constructing and validating the data collection tool; doing so is appropriate when the current study measures the same subjects, concepts, or traits as those measured by the existing tool.

Modifying an Existing Instrument. This approach can also provide some shortcuts in the process of developing the data collection tools. However, the researcher has to demonstrate the reasons for the modifications and document that these changes do not negatively affect the tool's reliability and validity. (See the section in this chapter about validity and reliability in quantitative research.)

Developing New Instruments. The third approach for developing tools specifically for the study is usually the most time-consuming and demanding; on the other hand, newly developed instruments tend to be most closely related to the study's specific purpose and research questions.

DATA COLLECTION PROCEDURES

The procedures used to collect data are described in this subsection. Information about how the study was conducted should be complete and clear enough to allow the study to be replicated. Information in this section may include the following: the process, duration, and schedule of the study, and a description of how the data were collected.

DATA ANALYSIS

This subsection describes how the data were analyzed, and the statistical tests used to analyze the data. The statistical tests may be listed in relation to the study's hypotheses. While this may be a helpful section, it is not always included in quantitative articles.

RESEARCH ETHICS

The rights and welfare of the study's participants should be assured; they should be informed of the nature of the research and be allowed to withdraw at any point. When minors participate in a study, their parents or legal guardians should provide their consent. Strictly following ethical guidelines is especially important in experimental studies where people participate in planned interventions (R. Ravid, 2015). In studies that involve human subjects, researchers should follow the guidelines provided by their professional associations, organizations, and/or universities.

Results

The findings from the study are presented in this section. If research questions and/ or hypotheses were stated for the study, they are repeated here and the data that were used to test them are presented. The main findings are reported and evaluated to determine whether they support the study's hypotheses. The results are presented here without an attempt to interpret them (McMillan & Wergin, 2010) or to offer explanations and implications. Numerical data, tables, and charts are often used to present the findings, along with a narrative that introduces and then interprets the data.

Discussion

The results are interpreted, evaluated, and explained in this section. When the results are unexpected or contrary to those predicted, tentative explanations should be provided (R. Ravid, 2015). This section also includes a discussion of how the study's findings fit with prior research on the topic, pointing to similarities, differences, and extensions of current knowledge.

Conclusions about the study and implications for practitioners are also found in this section. It is recommended that limitations of the current study and suggestions for future research be offered in the final discussion.

Validity and Reliability

In designing quantitative studies, researchers have to ensure the *external* and *internal validity* of their investigation. Internal validity refers to the degree that the researcher can demonstrate that the outcomes obtained are due to the planned intervention rather than extraneous variables that were not controlled in the study (R. Ravid, 2015); whereas external validity refers to the degree that the findings can be generalized to a larger population or to other settings.

Both types of validity are especially important in experimental research that investigates cause-and-effect relationships. Internal validity refers to the extent that researchers can document that any changes in the variable under study (dependent variable) were caused by the planned treatment (the independent variable) and not by other uncontrolled variables. Those uncontrolled or unanticipated variables (often referred to as extraneous variables) may present an alternative explanation for the study's outcomes (the dependent variable). (For more information, see *www.socialresearchmethods.net/kb/intval.php*). Threats to internal validity include bias in selecting the study participants (e.g., using volunteers for the experimental group), testing (the effect that a pretest has on the posttest performance of study participants), history (events that happen while the study takes place that may affect the dependent variable, especially in long-term studies), and instrumentation (the level of reliability and validity of the instrument being used to assess the effectiveness of the intervention) (R. Ravid, 2015).

Most studies are aimed at extending their findings to other similar settings, groups, and populations, rather than addressing only a local issue. Therefore, in order to contribute to the body of knowledge, a study should have high external validity, in addition to internal validity. There is, though, some tension between internal and external validity. In order to be of value, a study should have a tight control to ensure high internal validity; but this tight control makes the study unlike real life, thus limiting its external validity.

VALIDITY AND RELIABILITY OF DATA COLLECTION TOOLS

The validity of the data collection tools should also be reported. This type of validity refers to the extent to which an instrument measures that which it is designed to measure and whether appropriate inferences and interpretations are made using the results of the instrument (R. Ravid, 2015). It is important to remember that data collection tools are developed and validated for a specific purpose; thus, when they are used for other purposes or in different contexts, the validity has to be reestablished and documented.

There are three major types of validity that relate to data collection tools: (1) Content validity (whether the items or questions measure the content they are designed to measure); (2) criterion-related validity (whether the scores relate to another external tool that measures the same or related concepts); and (3) construct validity (whether the scores measure what they are supposed to measure) (Creswell & Plano Clark, 2011).

Reliability of data collection tools refers to the consistency and dependability of the instruments used to gather data (R. Ravid, 2015). There are several ways to assess the reliability of a measuring tool, and all of them rely on the use of correlation among the test items or with other quantitative measures (Mertler, 2012). Some of the most common ways of assessing reliability are (1) test–retest, where the same test is administered twice to the same group of examinees and the scores from the two testing sessions are correlated and compared; (2) alternate forms, in which two alternate forms of the same test are given to the same group of examinees and the scores of each person from the two testing sessions are correlated; (3) measures of internal consistency, which refers to using the scores from a single testing to assess the reliability of the whole test (R. Ravid, 2015).

Different types of studies require instruments with various levels of reliability. For example, the reliability of psychological tests used to diagnose and place people into treatment should have a reliability of .90 or higher. High-stakes achievement tests also commonly have reliabilities over .90. By comparison, lower levels of reliability are acceptable for measurement tools used in a study to assess a group of students, especially if they are used to measure noncognitive performances or traits.

When discussing the validity of an instrument, its reliability should also be reported because reliability is a precondition to validity. It is safe to expect that no measure is totally valid (Galvan & Galvan, 2017), but the assumption is that valid tests are also reliable.

TO DO: Quantitative Research Evaluation Checklist

To appraise quantitative studies, you may want to use the checklist in Table 6.2. This checklist provides a systematic way to identify the strengths and weaknesses of the methodology, results, discussion, and reliability and validity.

TABLE 6.2. A Checklist for Evaluating Quantitative Research Articles: Methodology, Results, Discussion, and Validity and Reliability

Quantitative research articles			✓
Methodology		▪ Description should be specific and detailed.	
		▪ Whether the study was experimental or nonexperimental is noted.	
	Participants	▪ There is a clear and detailed description of the participants and their characteristics.	
		▪ There is an explanation of how the sample was selected.	
	Data collection tools	▪ Data collection tools are clearly described.	
		▪ Information is provided as to whether existing, modified, or newly developed data collection tools are used.	
		▪ There is information about the reliability and validity of the data collection tools.	
		▪ When appropriate, sample items or questions are included.	
	Procedures	▪ The procedures for conducting the study are clearly and adequately described.	
		▪ There is a description of the process, duration, and schedule of the study.	
		▪ The data collection process is described.	
	Data analysis	▪ There is an explanation of the study's design and data analysis.	
		▪ Statistical procedures used to test the study's hypotheses are listed when appropriate.	

(continued)

TABLE 6.2. *(continued)*		
Quantitative research articles		✓
Ethics	▪ Ethical guidelines are followed.	
Results	▪ The main findings are reported.	
	▪ The results are clearly presented and easy to follow.	
	▪ There are tables, graphs, or charts that help explain the findings.	
Discussion	▪ The results are examined, explained, and evaluated.	
	▪ There is a discussion of the findings in relation to the original questions and/or hypotheses.	
	▪ Findings are discussed in relation to prior research on the topic.	
	▪ The study's conclusions are justified based on the results of the study.	
	▪ The authors provide possible explanations for unexpected results.	
	▪ Weaknesses and limitations of the study are discussed.	
	▪ Implications of the findings for practitioners are presented.	
	▪ There are suggestions for further research.	
Validity and Reliability	▪ There is evidence of the study's internal validity, especially in experimental studies.	
	▪ There is evidence of external validity.	
	▪ The validity of the data collection instrument(s) is presented.	
	▪ The reliability of the data collection instrument(s) is documented.	
	▪ The level of reliability of the measure is appropriate for its use in the study.	
	▪ The reliability levels of the data collection instrument(s) are reported when validity is discussed.	

Qualitative Research: Methodology, Ethical Considerations, Results, Discussion, Validity, and Trustworthiness

Methodology

The methodology section in qualitative studies follows a similar process as described above for quantitative research; however, qualitative inquiry typically tends to be holistic, subjective, and interpretative. These characteristics are mirrored in the methodology's strategies and procedures (Creswell, 2012). There are several approaches to qualitative research. Here we highlight the characteristics most common among them.

RESEARCHER'S ROLE

The researcher's subjectivity is acknowledged and perceived as a given in qualitative research. Self-awareness of one's values, assumptions, and biases is clearly and honestly stated. The researcher is thoughtful about his or her preconceived notions about the study's topic and practices disciplined subjectivity. This means an awareness of the impact of one's subjectivity, and an effort to monitor its influence on the study's process and findings (Marshall & Rossman, 2011).

SETTING

Qualitative research is embedded within particular settings and knowledge of the contextual factors of the research site is essential for a holistic understanding of the inquiry findings. The researcher should provide detailed information about the setting and offer a rationale for selecting it for the study.

PARTICIPANTS

Background information on the study's participants and a rationale for the sampling procedures should be offered. The sample in qualitative studies is selected purposively and deliberately and is based mostly on the participants' experiential knowledge about the topic and their ability and willingness to share it with the researcher (Efron & Ravid, 2013).

DATA COLLECTION TOOLS

Detailed information about the data collection tools and the rationale for choosing these particular strategies should be provided. The most common types of data collection strategies in qualitative studies are open-ended observations, interviews, documents, and audio and visual material. The Internet and social media have also become popular tools among qualitative researchers. Data collection often includes the use of multiple sources of data, thus enabling the researcher to *triangulate* the patterns and trends in the data collected and to corroborate the findings (Merriam, 2009).

PROCEDURES

In this section the researcher describes the research process and identifies the data collection and recording methods. Additionally, a record of the process is available (mostly in the appendices). This includes interview and observation protocols, field notes, transcripts, original and annotated documents, and informant consent (Bazeley, 2013).

DATA ANALYSIS

In this section the researcher usually describes the systematic process that is used for coding the data, identifying emerging categories, and synthesizing and interpreting the discovered patterns. The researcher uses evidence to support the findings, searches for alternative interpretations, and employs different sources to triangulate his or her assertions, thus enhancing the trustworthiness of the findings. The researcher also reflects on whether disciplined subjectivity was practiced and ensures that preconceived assumptions do not color the interpretation (Richards, 2009).

Ethical Considerations

In most qualitative studies there is direct interaction with the participants during the data collection process. Since it is not feasible to assure the anonymity of the participants, there is a special need to protect their confidentiality, interest, and well-being. The researcher should ensure that the participants and the setting's identity are not revealed by name or with identifying information. Participants have to be notified regarding the nature and the goals of the study and they should consent in writing to take part in it. When the participants are minors, their parents or guardians should sign a consent form. Formal ethical permission to conduct the study should be obtained from the appropriate bodies (Miller & Birch, 2012).

Results

The study's findings may be organized thematically around the categories, themes, and patterns, or by a chronological description of the study process. Reporting on the results is done in what qualitative researchers describe as a "thick" narrative (i.e., a rich, detailed, and vivid account). The findings are supported by evidence from the data, quotations from participants' perspectives in their own voices, as well as detailed descriptions of contexts, events, actions, interactions, and participants' behavior. The findings may also be contextualized within theoretical frameworks and linked to the literature on the topic (Yin, 2015).

Discussion

In this final section of the study, the researcher discusses holistically the meaning of the findings. Meaning is discussed in relation to the research question(s). There may also be considerations of the findings' implications and the actions they invoke. While qualitative studies usually limit the implications of the results to the setting of the study, the conclusions may lead to a transferability of the findings to other similar contexts. Additionally, the interpretation of the study's findings may lead to a discussion of the phenomenon within broader social, cultural, and political contexts (Maxwell, 2013). The researcher often adds a personal reflection about the study process from his or her perspective.

Validity and Trustworthiness

Most qualitative researchers agree that qualitative studies should not be judged against standards borrowed from quantitative approaches but rather on the basis of criteria that reflect the unique nature of this approach. Lincoln and Guba (1985), in their seminal book, proposed a set of guidelines to establish the trustworthiness of qualitative studies and to define the concept of validity and reliability within a qualitative research framework. These guidelines are comprised of four criteria: credibility, transferability, dependability, and conformability.

> ▶ *Credibility* focuses on the accuracy and integrity of a study, and the believability of its findings.
> ▶ *Transferability* examines whether the study results may be applied to another comparable setting where a similar research question is examined.
> ▶ *Dependability* assesses whether the procedures used during the inquiry are appropriate for the study's question(s) and were adequately implemented.
> ▶ *Conformability* considers the extent to which the study's findings represent the data accurately rather than reflect the researcher's bias.

When the quality of a qualitative study and the trustworthiness of its findings are appraised, attention should be given to the following issues that are drawn from the four criteria listed above (Bazeley, 2013; Creswell, 2012; Galvan, 2014; Marshall & Rossman, 2011; Maxwell, 2013).

Drawing from the four criteria above, researchers (e.g., Bazeley, 2013; Creswell, 2012; Galvan & Galvan, 2017; Marshall & Rossman, 2011; Maxwell, 2013) suggest the following benchmarks to appraise the strength of a qualitative study and to evaluate the trustworthiness of its findings:

> ▶ *Prolonged engagement* in the research setting allows an in-depth understanding of the study's setting and participants. It strengthens the researcher's insight into the participants' culture, perspectives, behavior, and interactions.
> ▶ *Researcher bias* should be openly and honestly discussed throughout the research process. The researcher's subjectivity should be monitored and kept in check through self-reflection. Information about personal and professional involvement with the topic and the participants should be disclosed.

▶ *Description of the research process and procedures* used in the study should be explicit and detailed. To demonstrate that these procedures were adequate, the researcher should describe the inquiry process and include details about the sample selection, the data collection and analysis tools, and the rationale for choosing them.

▶ *Thick description* should be provided as part of the analysis section. This includes vivid descriptions of the context, the events, and the participants. Additionally, quotations that capture the participants' points of view and their experiences, as seen from their perspectives, should be interwoven throughout the narrative.

▶ *Triangulation* of data obtained from multiple sources should be utilized. This is done in order to corroborate the information, cross-examine the identified patterns and trends, and strengthen the credibility of the findings discovered in the data.

▶ *Negative case analysis* of alternative possible interpretation and discrepant information should be presented. The researcher should relate the strategies used to check possible counter-understandings and how they were taken into account as the study findings were interpreted.

▶ *Member checking* should be used to ensure that the participants' perspectives and experiences are accurately presented in the research narrative. The transcripts, the data analysis, and the final findings may be shared with the participants to enhance accuracy.

▶ *Peer debriefing* refers to sharing the study with other researchers in order to ascertain the credibility and trustworthiness of the process used in conducting the research.

TO DO: *Qualitative Research Evaluation Checklist*

To appraise qualitative studies, you may want to use the checklist in Table 6.3 (pp. 111–112). This checklist provides a systematic way to identify the strengths or weaknesses of the methodology, results, discussion, and validity and trustworthiness found in published qualitative studies.

TABLE 6.3. A Checklist for Evaluating Qualitative Research Articles: Methodology, Results, Discussion, and Validity and Trustworthiness

Qualitative research articles			✓
Methodology	▣ Description should be specific and detailed.		
	Researcher's role	▣ Researcher's subjectivity and preconceived notions about the topic are discussed.	
	Setting	▣ Detailed information about the setting and rationale for selecting it is provided.	
	Participants	▣ Background information about the participants is offered.	
		▣ Participant selection is based on their knowledge of the topic and their ability and willingness to share it.	
	Data collection tools	▣ The process of data collection is clearly and comprehensively described.	
		▣ Methods used to generate data are clearly described.	
		▣ Multiple sources of data collection were used to enable triangulation.	
		▣ Data collection strategies are appropriate for the research question(s).	
	Procedures	▣ The procedures for conducting the study are clearly and adequately described.	
		▣ A record of the process, including interviews, observations, protocols, field notes, and transcripts, is available in the appendix.	
	Data analysis	▣ The method of data analysis is logically developed and clearly presented.	
		▣ The process for coding the data and for identifying categories, themes, and patterns is outlined.	
		▣ The relationships among the patterns are supported by the data.	
	Ethics	▣ The identity of the participants and the settings is kept confidential.	
		▣ Formal ethical permissions to conduct the study were obtained.	
		▣ The participants were informed about the nature of the research and their confidentiality was assured.	
Results	▣ There is a clear explanation of how the findings are drawn from the data analysis.		
	▣ The results are reported in a "thick" narrative.		
	▣ The findings are supported by illustrative quotations and specific instances.		
	▣ The findings clearly and adequately address the research question(s).		
	▣ Contradictory findings and outlier data are included in the research findings.		

(continued)

TABLE 6.3. *(continued)*		
Qualitative research articles		✓
Discussion	▪ The meaning and implications of the study are discussed in relation to the research questions.	
	▪ The discussion relates the study's findings to existing literature on the topic.	
	▪ The findings are discussed within the broader social, cultural, and/or political contexts.	
	▪ The researcher reflects on the experiences of conducting the study.	
Validity and Trustworthiness	▪ The credibility, transferability, dependability, and conformability of the study are discussed.	
	▪ The research process and data collection phases entailed a prolonged engagement.	
	▪ The researcher discusses personal biases and preconceived assumptions.	
	▪ The research process, procedures, and documentation are recorded.	
	▪ There is a rich ("thick") description of the participants, the setting(s), and the events.	
	▪ There is an explanation on how data results were triangulated.	
	▪ Processes for alternative possible interpretation and discrepant information are presented.	
	▪ Procedures for checking the research accuracy from the perspective of participants and peer researchers are used.	

Mixed-Methods Research: Methodology, Results, Discussion, Validity, Reliability, and Trustworthiness

Methodology

Mixed-methods research refers to the blending or combining of quantitative and qualitative methods and techniques into a single study. The two methods are blended in studies where researchers believe that data collection using only one approach is not sufficient (Creswell & Plano Clark, 2011). The order and importance of the quantitative and qualitative methods can differ from study to study reflecting the research design used. Three common types of mixed-methods designs are: (1) embedded design, (2) two-phase design, and (3) triangulation design (Efron & Ravid, 2013). The researchers should clearly explain the reasons for choosing to use multiple methods and how they were implemented in the study. Mixed-methods research presents quantitative and qualitative questions and the chosen methods should match those questions.

RESEARCHER'S ROLE

The researcher assumes an objective or subjective stance or attitude depending on the research question under investigation.

SETTING AND PARTICIPANTS

As was described when discussing the quantities and qualitative approaches, the reasons for selecting the sample, the type of sample selected, the characteristics of the participants, and the setting where the study was conducted should be clearly described.

DATA COLLECTION TOOLS

Both quantitative and qualitative data collection tools should be described in this section. The description should be detailed and specific enough to allow readers to duplicate the study, if they choose to do so. Sample questions or items should also be included.

PROCEDURES

The data collection strategies can be used either simultaneously or sequentially. The different data tools complement each other by highlighting different aspects of the same questions (Efron & Ravid, 2013). The steps used to collect both quantitative and qualitative data should be explicitly described.

DATA ANALYSIS

The procedures for data analysis vary among the three types of mixed- methods designs (embedded, two-phased, and triangulation). The differences are based on three elements: (1) whether the data are analyzed sequentially or concurrently, (2) how and when the integration of the quantitative and qualitative data occur, and (3) whether the quantitative or qualitative approach is given priority in the study or the two approaches are equal (Creswell, 2018).

Results

In mixed-methods studies, the results from the quantitative phase allow the researcher to inform, strengthen, and explain the findings from the qualitative phase; and the findings from the qualitative phase allow the researcher to further explain the results from the quantitative phase. The data can also be mixed, as in triangulation design, where both quantitative and qualitative findings are integrated and analyzed concurrently (McMillan & Schumacher, 2010).

Results are presented in different formats based on the data source that yielded these findings. The conventions described in this chapter for presenting the results from quantitative and qualitative data sources apply in mixed-methods studies as well. An explanation should be given of how the findings from the quantitative and qualitative methods were integrated.

Ethical Considerations

The ethical considerations listed for quantitative and qualitative studies should be followed in mixed-methods research as well.

Discussion

Reporting the study's conclusions and their meaning does not differ a great deal when writing quantitative, qualitative, or mixed-methods studies. All research reports present, interpret, and explain results. Findings should be evaluated in light of other research reported in the literature review. If there are conflicting findings due to the use of different research methods, they are examined and properly explained. Limitations and suggestions for further research should also be offered.

Validity, Reliability, and Trustworthiness of Mixed-Methods Studies

The procedures for ensuring the validity, reliability, and trustworthiness of mixed-methods research reflect the specific requirements of each approach. Therefore, when appraising mixed-methods research researchers should follow the guidelines for quantitative and qualitative approaches described in this chapter.

TO DO: ***Mixed-Methods Research Evaluation Checklist***

To assess the quality of mixed-methods studies you may want to use the checklist in Table 6.4. This checklist provides a systematic way to identify the strengths or weaknesses of the methodology, results, discussion, validity, reliability, and trustworthiness found in published mixed-methods studies. (For further details on how to assess quantitative and qualitative studies see Tables 6.2 and 6.3.)

TABLE 6.4. A Checklist for Evaluating Mixed-Methods Research Articles: Methodology, Results, Discussion, and Validity, Reliability, and Trustworthiness			
Mixed-methods research articles			✓
Methodology	▪ The reasons for choosing a mixed-methods approach are clearly explained.		
	▪ The methods used match the research questions, and each method is designed to answer at least one research question.		
	Researcher's role	▪ The researcher role—an objective or subjective stance—is assumed to match the research question being investigated.	
	Site and participants	▪ The site and participants are fully described and the reasons for selecting them are presented.	
			(continued)

TABLE 6.4. *(continued)*			
Mixed-methods research articles			✓
Methodology *(continued)*	**Data collection tools**	▪ Data collection tools, both quantitative and qualitative, are described in detail.	
		▪ Sample items from data collection tools are included.	
	Procedures	▪ The steps used to collect both quantitative and qualitative data are explicitly described.	
	Data analysis	▪ The procedures for data analysis reflect the type of mixed data designs (embedded, two-phased, or triangulation).	
		▪ It is indicated whether the analysis occurred sequentially or concurrently.	
		▪ It is indicated when the integration of quantitative and qualitative data occurred.	
		▪ It is clear whether the quantitative or qualitative approach is given priority.	
	Ethics	▪ The ethical considerations listed for quantitative and qualitative studies are followed.	
Results		▪ Findings are presented in different formats based on the method and data source used to generate the data.	
		▪ An explanation is offered of how findings from the quantitative and qualitative methods are integrated.	
Discussion		▪ The major findings are reiterated in relation to the study's questions.	
		▪ Conflicting findings are examined and properly explained.	
		▪ The study's findings are evaluated in relation to prior research in the field.	
Validity, reliability, and trustworthiness		▪ The procedures for ensuring the validity, reliability, and trustworthiness of mixed-methods research follow the specific requirements of each approach.	

HERMENEUTIC–PHENOMENOLOGICAL RESEARCH: ORIENTATION, DEPTH, STRENGTH, AND RICHNESS

Broadly speaking, hermeneutics is the theory and methodology of interpreting text. Inquiries written in this tradition are mainly used in philosophical and conceptual studies that focus on understanding texts through interpretation and reflective deliberation. The researcher's data may include philosophical or theoretical narrative, poetry, fiction, and anything else that provokes thinking (Smythe & Spence, 2012). According to Max van Manen (2014), "To write is to reflect; to write is to research" (p. 20). The writers do not report the content of the text but rather focus on its meaning (Smith, 1991). Hermeneutic researchers interpret the writings on their topic "so that the work of others turns into a conversation partnership that reveals the limits and possibilities of one's own interpretive achievements" (van Manen, 1990, p. 76). This approach to research resists offering a single authoritative reading of the text and embraces the idea that the same text may present itself in numerous meaningful ways (Gadamer, 2004).

The ambiguous nature of the hermeneutic tradition does not lend itself to unanimous criteria of quality appraisal (Gadamer, 2004). Still, hermeneutic researchers assert that there are a number of requirements that need to be attended to in a rigorous study (Smith, 1999). The following evaluative criteria, based on van Manen's (1990, pp. 151–152) suggestions, are *orientation, depth, strength,* and *richness*.

Orientation

Hermeneutic researchers do not report on the content of the reviewed texts but rather interpret the texts with a focus on their meaning. This meaning is drawn from the involvement of the researcher in the world of the participants and their stories (Kafle, 2011). It is accepted that since the researchers are closely involved with the researched texts, their predispositions are an integral part of the meaning they make of it. Thus, the text interpretation draws from the researchers' subjective horizon of understanding (van Manen, 1990), which means their particular biographies, values, preconceptions, and prejudices. This subjectivity also includes the writer's perspective on the historical, political, and cultural background that surrounds the topic. This subjectivity serves as a backdrop for the researcher's meaning-making and it cannot be avoided.

Writers should be attentive to the multiple levels of subjectivity and biases they brings to their interpretations, openly acknowledge them, and contemplate their impact throughout the writing process (Gadamer, 2004; Van Manen, 1990). Although their interpretations, insights, and the meaning they make reflect their subjective positions, those positions should be supported with a rich analysis of relevant references.

Depth

Researchers should not be satisfied in mirroring themselves in the texts, but rather be open to different perspectives and orientations. The purpose is not to undermine one's subjectivity, but to deepen and expand existing horizons by drawing from a broad range of relevant research across time, cultures, and contexts. The depth of the article is expressed in the ability of the writer to enter into the participants' lived worlds and convey their intentions (Kafle, 2011). These intentions are presented within the context of similar, diverse, or opposing points of view.

The narrative is presented in a dialogical style and the researchers are engaged in conversations with authors holding different perspectives. The dialogical encounters provoke new understandings that go beyond the taken-for-granted assumptions (Barrett, Powley, & Pearce, 2011) and lead to "new ways of seeing and thinking within a deep sense of tradition" (Smith, 1991, p. 202).

Strength

Researchers should describe the philosophical underpinnings of the hermeneutic approach. They should consider the reasons for choosing this particular perspective and how this tradition of research complements the aims and objectives of their work.

Hermeneutic researchers should be able to present their understanding of the inherent meanings revealed through the participants' stories and narrative. According to the hermeneutic tradition, the strength of the interpretation is enhanced when it is done within the cultural and historical background of texts. The researchers should consider the effects of these contexts on the authors they discuss and highlight the philosophical frames of reference that undergird these writers' ideas and concepts.

Hermeneutic writers should maintain a balance between an understanding of the broad context and the interpretation of a specific text (Gadamer, 2004). There should be a back-and-forth circular movement between the whole (context) and the part (particular text) in a continuous dialogue "in such a way as to bring both into view simultaneously" (Geertz, 1979, p. 23).

Richness

Hermeneutic researchers reflect on the relationship between the form and the content of the narrative and pay close attention to the evocative power of language usage (van Manen, 2014). The etymological roots of words and tracing their historical meaning, as well as their current connotations, are valuable in this research tradition. Additionally, following the tradition of intense aesthetic quality (Ricoeur, 1981), the narrative of the literature review should be creative, original, and rich (Langdridge, 2007). The lingual deliberation in terms of metaphors, poetic images, similes, and analogies helps generate new insights and bring to the surface the multiple meanings of the text (Ricoeur, 1981; van Manen, 2014).

Paying attention to the language also entails clear, lucid, engaging, and persuasive writing. The arguments are well organized and the thoughts, concepts, and insights flow coherently. The concepts and assertions are developed on the basis of a logical chain of reasoning, the ideas and insights of the reviewed authors are thoughtfully discussed, and the conclusions flow reasonably from the conceptual and philosophical deliberations.

Finally, richness in hermeneutic research also means that the writing provokes new understanding and insights about the topic at the center of the review. The writer invites the reader to take part in the dialogue among the writers that are reviewed, to contemplate the thoughts and comprehensions surfaced through the discussion, and to continue the conversation.

TO DO: Hermeneutic–Phenomenological Research Articles Evaluation Checklist

To assess the quality of hermeneutic–phenomenological research texts you may want to use the checklist in Table 6.5. This checklist provides a systematic way to appraise the quality of the text based on the criteria offered by van Manen (1990).

TABLE 6.5. A Checklist for Evaluating Hermeneutic–Phenomenological Research Articles Using van Manen's Criteria

Hermeneutic–phenomenological research articles		✓
Orientation	▪ The researcher interprets the texts with a focus on their meaning rather than merely reporting on them.	
	▪ The interpretation reflects the researcher's biography, values, and prejudices.	
	▪ The researcher is mindful of his or her perspective on the historical, political, and cultural background surrounding the topic.	
	▪ The researcher reveals his or her biases and prejudices and reflects on how they shape the meanings given to the texts.	
Depth	▪ The sources that the writer reflects on are presented within the context of similar, diverse, or opposing points of view.	
	▪ The writer draws from a broad range of relevant research across time, cultures, and contexts.	
	▪ The narrative is presented in a dialogical style and the researcher is engaged in conversations with different authors' perspectives.	
	▪ The author presents an understanding that goes beyond the taken-for-granted assumptions on a subject.	

(continued)

TABLE 6.5. *(continued)*		✓
Hermeneutic–phenomenological research articles		
Strength	◼ The researcher discusses the tradition of hermeneutic–phenomenological philosophy that underpins the research.	
	◼ The writer explains why this type of review was chosen and how it complements the research aims and objectives.	
	◼ The researcher discusses the effects of the contextual background on the writings of the authors reviewed.	
	◼ The researcher presents the philosophical and theoretical perspectives of the studies discussed.	
	◼ The writer maintains a balance between an understanding of the broad context and the interpretation of a specific text.	
Richness	◼ The researcher reflects on the relationship between the form and the content of the narrative.	
	◼ The writer explores the hidden meaning of language by tracing its historical and etymological roots, as well as its current connotations.	
	◼ The researcher's narrative style is creative and uses poetic images, metaphors, similes, and so forth.	
	◼ The narrative is clear, coherent, engaging, and persuasive.	
	◼ The narrative provokes new understanding and insights about the topic.	

GROUP WORK

1. Choose two articles representing two of the research types discussed in this chapter (quantitative, qualitative, mixed methods, and hermeneutic–phenomenological).
2. Using the criteria checklist(s) for these two types, assess the quality of the selected articles.
3. Share your assessment with your group, highlighting the points that are most relevant for your literature review.

WHAT'S NEXT?

This chapter explored the value of a critical evaluation of the literature you review and presented criteria that may serve to assess your sources. The next chapter focuses on building a logical structure of your review of the literature by developing organizational strategies that allow your review to flow logically and smoothly from one argument to the next.

CHAPTER SUMMARY

1. When you write a literature review, it is important that you adopt a critical stance toward the sources you review and acknowledge their weaknesses, as well as their strengths.

2. Rather than critique each article on its own, it might, at times, be better to critique groups of sources together, especially when you identify a pattern of weakness that is common across these studies.

3. All types of research draw their quality standards out of their traditions, orientations, expectations, and norms.

4. There are sections in articles that are common to quantitative, qualitative, mixed-methods, and hermeneutic–phenomenological research. These sections are the title, abstract, introduction, and literature review.

5. To ensure the ethics of quantitative, qualitative, and mixed-methods research, the rights and welfare of the study's participants should be assured. They should be informed of the nature of the research and be allowed to withdraw at any point.

6. In designing quantitative studies, researchers have to ensure the *external* validity and *internal* validity of their investigation.

7. There are three positions regarding the value of assessing qualitative research: (a) the criteria used by quantitative researchers should be applied equally to qualitative studies; (b) a unique set of criteria should be used to assess qualitative research; and (c) a rejection of any kind of criteria in assessing qualitative research.

8. The sections commonly found in the methodology section of qualitative studies are researcher role, setting, participants, data collection tools, procedures, and data analysis. These sections should provide detailed information for readers to gain a holistic understanding of the research process.

9. Mixed-methods research presents quantitative and qualitative questions and, depending on the question, the chosen methods for data collection, analysis, and interpretation should reflect both approaches.

10. The ambiguous nature of hermeneutic–phenomenological tradition does not lend itself to unanimous criteria of quality appraisal. However, four evaluative criteria are often used by researchers: *orientation, depth, strength,* and *richness.*

CHAPTER 7

Structuring and Organizing the Literature Review

By now you have summarized, analyzed, and assessed individual studies, articles, and books, as well as identified some of the core terms, central concepts, and methodologies that are relevant to your topic. Now you are ready to assemble the individual pieces of information and weave them together into a holistic narrative. A major goal of literature review writers is to demonstrate comprehensive understanding and insight into the current state of knowledge on their chosen topic. This goal cannot be achieved through a series of summaries of individual sources that are patched together one by one. Rather, the aim is to develop a holistic narrative that is analyzed, synthesized, and organized thoughtfully and logically. The theories, research methodologies, and findings extracted from the literature should be woven together to reveal patterns, discover relationships, and build a logical chain of claims supported by data.

Like a jigsaw puzzle in which the individual pieces are put together to reveal the whole picture, a review requires you to assemble the literature's various threads in a way that allows readers to gain "a bird's-eye view, or even better, a series of bird's-eye views" (Feak & Swales, 2009, p. 17). This process of reassembling should not be a patchwork, but rather be built around a logical structure where the data, theories, claims, and arguments present the "big picture" of up-to-date knowledge about your research topic and research question. At the same time, your review should also provoke new thinking and understanding through fresh and creative connections that you have captured within and among the different concepts, theories, and research.

To unearth a meaningful storyline in your literature review without getting lost in the details, you need to develop an organizational strategy. This will help you in several ways. It will impose logical order on your multiple sources, enhance your understanding of the body of knowledge relevant to your topic, and advance the development of a new perspective on the literature. Thus, an organizational design serves as the blueprint that will assist you in structuring the rich material you have gathered, highlight common themes among the different studies, compare and contrast the findings, and discern common and unusual patterns. Such an architectural plan will also allow the presentation of your ideas to flow logically and smoothly from one argument to the next.

There is no one uniform organizational strategy for structuring the literature review that allows you to make connections, highlight relationships, and bring coherence to the different individual studies (Ridley, 2012). However, there are several methods that are used by researchers to synthesize the information into an organized whole. In this chapter we describe the four approaches most often used by literature review writers: synthesis matrix, summary table, mapping, and outline. These strategies are different from each other in their organization techniques, formats of presentation, and the aspects of structure that they highlight. Each strategy contributes in different ways to your ability to identify themes and patterns in your sources, determine how they relate to each other, and discern the similarities and differences among them.

APPROACHES TO ORGANIZING THE LITERATURE REVIEW

Like other literature review writers, you have to discover the organizational strategy that works best for you. Being aware of your own style of writing will help you choose the strategy that will benefit you the most. Your choice of organizational strategy also depends on the research question(s) undergirding your review and how you want to present your knowledge in response to this question.

Some writers prefer formulating their organization device early in the literature review process, while others favor doing it at a more advanced stage, after they have explored the research articles for some time (Ridley, 2012). The needs at each stage may be different and the strategy you choose will probably reflect that. However, as Ridley suggests, whatever strategy you decide to use, expect it to change or even be replaced as your work progresses. Moreover, the organizational structure that seems so logical at one point may evolve and transform as you advance with your reading and deepen your understanding of the issues discussed in the review.

In any case, before you create the organizational structure, you may want to revisit your research question and determine whether it still reflects your focus or needs to be revised. Your question has a major role in developing the organizational structure of the literature review analysis and synthesis, so be sure that it still reflects your purpose for writing your review.

Next, we describe the four literature review organizational strategies mentioned above. We define and highlight what distinguishes each, examine their advantages, describe how to construct them, and offer examples that illustrate how they may be used.

THE SYNTHESIS MATRIX

The synthesis matrix strategy involves an iterative process where you examine your analysis of individual sources and cluster them together in a grid to discern patterns and themes in the literature (Whittemore & Knafl, 2005). This strategy facilitates your ability to systematically compare authors' different perspectives, studies' methodologies, and findings and see the relationships among them (Garrard, 2014). Thus, the synthesis matrix enables you to achieve an overview of the literature, helps you identify relationships and pattern, and provides a succinct organization that gathers related ideas, issues, or results under broader topical themes and subthemes. A synthesis matrix can serve as an organizational strategy on its own or be used as a baseline for other strategic organizational approaches, such as mapping or outline. (Helpful tools for creating the synthesis matrix are article note-taking index cards [ANTICs], as well as the thematic concentric circles; both are described in Chapter 5.)

How to Construct the Synthesis Matrix
The list in Table 7.1 outlines the steps involved in creating a synthesis matrix.

TABLE 7.1. Steps for Creating a Synthesis Matrix
Step
1. Go back to the notes you have taken in the ANTIC for each literature source. Look for the key concepts or keywords you have identified on each index card, and the accompanying entries in which you analyzed and summarized the key relevant concepts that were discussed in that source.
2. Comb the rest of the ANTICs and look for the same keywords or concepts. Be careful not to miss any relevant source; you may have named similar or related issues or concepts with different keywords.
3. Once you have identified the related notes, group them near one another in a grid. Be sure to note the reference for each entry.

(continued)

TABLE 7.1. *(continued)*

Step

4. The process of clustering these sections within the individual index cards can be done by cutting and pasting (with the use of a word-processing system) or it can be facilitated with the use of computer software programs. Digital notebooks such as Evernote, One Note, and Workflow are effective in locating and retrieving keywords within the index cards' entries (Garrard, 2014).

5. Review the clustered notes and through an iterative process try to discern patterns, common and repeating issues, and topical themes. Look for similarities among these entries and see how they relate to one another and how they are logically connected. Label the group of notes with an identifying name that reflects an emerging, connecting theme (Whittemore & Knafl, 2005). Remember, a theme is a broad, more encompassing concept that contains subthemes, related ideas, common arguments or findings. For example, the theme of *assessment* may include types of assessment, use of assessments, and debates about assessment.

6. Write a short reflection in which you respond to the entry, compare it to other sources, and highlight points you want to consider or want to explore further. For example, as you read an article on assessment, you may want to write a note to find additional articles that investigate the history of assessment.

7. Compare and contrast the notes that you clustered under each theme. A theme doesn't mean that the studies comprise a unified perspective or single methodology. Rather, a theme includes agreeing with or complementing, as well as contradicting, positions held by researchers and theoreticians who have explored the same issue. For example, within the theme of assessment the writer may review studies whose authors are proponents of the use of standardized tests for evidence-based decision making in education. On the other hand, it may include studies conducted by researchers who criticize the overuse of standardized tests for accountability and instead support the use of teacher-made tests for making local educational decisions.

8. You may organize the individual entries within each theme into subgroups according to a coherent and logical order. You may arrange these subgroups in several ways. For example, sequentially, according to the type of methodology used, or structure them from general to more particular information. In another example, when you locate a seminal study, you may want to arrange research published after that study in chronological order (Garrard, 2014). Later in this chapter we consider how themes may be organized.

9. Revisit and refine the emerging themes. See if all the studies belong under this theme or if there is research that should form another theme or be discarded altogether (Garrard, 2014).

The development of the synthesis matrix is tentative and iterative and may evolve throughout the process. The emerging patterns and themes may not be clearly observable until you obtain a fuller picture of the literature on your topic. Additionally, in the early phase of the review process you will probably not fill all the spaces in the matrix. As you continue reading and adding ANTICs, you will be able to refine the themes: insert additional entries as well as themes and subthemes, combine some into one, or rearrange the order of the subgroups within the themes.

The final set of patterns, themes, and subthemes may not be completely established until the end of the process. Still, we suggest that from the earliest stages of the literature review you gradually develop the synthesis matrix and insert relevant information into the appropriate spaces. Doing so will help you gradually identify the emerging arguments and claims, and eventually identify the organizational scheme that will structure your literature review writing.

An Example of a Synthesis Matrix

To illustrate how to use a synthesis matrix, we present the matrix developed by Marina, who is writing the literature review chapter of her dissertation on the topic of mentoring in schools. Table 7.2 illustrates an early stage in the development of her matrix.

TABLE 7.2. An Example of an Early Phase in Building a Synthesis Matrix: Mentors' Roles and Practices

Themes and subthemes	Reference	Analysis and summary	Reflection/response
Definition of mentorship	Ambrosetti, A., & Dekkers, J. (2010). The interconnectedness of the role of mentors and mentees in pre-service teacher education. *Australian Journal of Teacher Education, 35*(6), 42–55.	The definition of mentoring is interconnected with the contextual factors that influence mentoring in teacher education. However, although there are numerous definitions, they do not clearly outline the actions that occur during the mentoring process. The authors' definition highlights the hierarchical and reciprocal relationships between the mentor and the mentee, who work together toward a defined outcome for the mentorship. Some other definitions of mentoring are: Mentoring is a process (Smith, 2007). Mentoring is a process but also a relationship (Kwan & Lopez-Real, 2005). Mentoring is contextual (Fairbank et al., 2000). Mentoring is relational, developmental, and contextual (Lai, 2005). **Quotation** (p. 52): "The relationship usually follows a developmental pattern within a specific timeframe and roles as defined, expectations are outlined and purpose is ideally clearly delineated."	Need to find the etymological source of the word "mentor" and its implication for current definitions. I like the assertion that the definition is part of the contextual factors. Need to expand this idea in my literature review chapter. I need to read the original articles which were noted in my summary. **Assessment:** A very comprehensive critical review of research literature on mentoring that consists of multiple sources. The article presents various definitions of mentoring currently used. It insightfully interprets how these definitions impact the way the mentors are perceived and what is expected of them by teachers, administrators, and researchers. No explanation is offered of how the sources were identified and what the inclusion and exclusion criteria were.

(continued)

TABLE 7.2. *(continued)*

Themes and subthemes	Reference	Analysis and summary	Reflection/response
Definition of mentorship *(continued)*	**Definition (etymological)** Online Etymology Dictionary *www.etymonline.com/ index.php?term=mentor*	"Wise adviser," from Greek: Mentor, friend of Odysseus and adviser of Telemachus. Mentor in the *Odyssey* means "adviser." "Intent, purpose, spirit, passion" from *mon-eyo- (cognates: Sanskrit man-tar- ["one who thinks"], Latin mon-i-tor ["one who admonishes"]), causative form of root *men- ("to think").	The fact that in the etymological source mentor was a wise "friend" emphasizes the equal relationship between mentor and mentee. The "thinking" aspect is an essential characteristic of the mentor. Thinking with or thinking for? This reflects two conflicting perceptions of the role.
	Hudson, P., & Hudson, S. (2010). Mentor educators' understanding of mentoring preservice primary teachers. *International Journal of Learning, 17*(2), 157–170.	Arriving at a common definition will assist the mentoring process. Clear communication among all parties involved will enhance their ability to share a common language when it comes to the role and responsibilities of the mentor. The common definition they used was "an experienced teacher who supports, influences, encourages, and challenges a mentee toward teaching competencies" (p. 165). The qualities of the mentor according to this definition are, among others, being supportive, facilitating reflection, possessing listening skills, and responding to professional needs.	Look for other articles that discuss definitions of mentors' roles to see if there is a connection between the definitions and how the roles are perceived by mentors and mentees
Mentor roles	Brondyk, S., & Searby, L. (2013). Best practice in mentoring: Complexities and possibilities. *Journal of Mentoring and Coaching in Education, 2*(3), 189–203.	The article highlights the many different roles that are involved in mentoring in primary and secondary schools. The authors note that the role of mentor may be viewed in three main ways: **Traditional:** Mentor as transmitter/messenger. Skills are transferred within an authoritative framework and within status quo culture. **Transitional:** Mentor as collaborator; mentor and mentee are co-learners. Cultural gaps are bridged and cultural differences are honored. **Transformational:** Mentor as change agent. Mentors and mentees are engaged in innovative and creative discourse. Their roles are fluid and changing. New realities are created as they engage in collective actions to transform the organization.	The three perceptions of the mentor roles remind me of Kent's (2013) article. Make a connection between the mentor's role and the context's expectations (Kent). **Assessment:** A conceptual paper. Thoughtful with many research citations to support the claim that it is difficult to identify best practice in mentoring because the mentoring process is so complex.

(continued)

TABLE 7.2. *(continued)*			
Themes and subthemes	**Reference**	**Analysis and summary**	**Reflection/response**
Mentor roles *(continued)*	Ambrosetti, A., & Dekkers, J. (2010). The interconnectedness of the role of mentors and mentees in pre-service teacher education, *Australian Journal of Teacher Education, 35*(6), 42–55.	Based on multiple articles, the authors present a list of common perceptions of the mentor roles: **Supporter:** Assists the mentee to grow personally and professionally. **Role model:** Assists by example and demonstration of desired behavior. **Facilitator:** Provides opportunities to mentees to grow by performing their tasks. **Assessor:** Assesses the mentee's performance and offers critique. **Collaborator:** Shares and reflects with the mentee in a collaborative relationship. **Friend:** Behaves as a critical friend. **Trainer:** Provides skills and resources. **Protector:** Protects the mentee from unpleasant situations. **Colleague:** Treats the mentee as an equal professional.	Interesting list. May be helpful in categorizing the mentors observed. Will I be able to group under the three perspectives suggested by S. Brondyk and L. Searby (2013)?
Mentor roles (From the perspective of acting mentors)	Hall, K. M., Draper, R. J., Smith, L. K., & Bullough, R. V. (2008). More than a place to teach: Exploring the perception of the roles and responsibilities. *Mentoring and Tutoring: Partnership in Learning, 16*(3), 328–345.	Mentors' perceptions of their role is influenced by the experiences they have had. The authors divide mentor roles into three groups: **Support provider:** Giving feedback, guiding, sharing ideas, and modeling. **Critical evaluator:** Giving constructive criticism with an emphasis on reflection and problem solving. **Team teaching:** Collaborating, planning activities, and teaching together as a team. Data based on open-ended survey given to 264 participants who are mentoring preservice teachers. The survey was followed with 34 phone interviews with randomly selected mentors.	The roles described here can be compared and contrasted to the roles discussed in other articles. Well-planned survey. May serve as a model for my research design.

(continued)

TABLE 7.2. *(continued)*

Themes and subthemes	Reference	Analysis and summary	Reflection/response
Effective mentoring practices (component of effective mentoring relationships)	Hudson, P., & Hudson, S. (2010). Mentor educators' understanding of mentoring preservice primary teachers. *The International Journal of Learning 17*(2), 157–170.	A mixed-methods study that focused on mentors' perspectives. The study involved surveys, questionnaires, and audiotaped focus group—14 mentors (4 m, 10 f) working with preservice teachers. From the mentors' perspective, three requirements were needed to form an effective mentoring experience: (a) knowing the mentor's level of development and expectations so the mentor can adequately support and challenge the mentee; (b) building professional relationships prior to placement—time is needed to establish the relationship and troubleshoot potential problems; and (c) dual role as confidant and assessor: neither role can be discounted. Mentor as confidant allows the mentor to build self-confidence and experiment with practice, while mentor as assessor can be used to guide the teacher's growth.	**Consideration:** The idea of mentee's developmental stage should be expanded in my paper. **Critique:** Very detailed analysis and results section. A bit confusing in highlighting the major themes.
	Efron, E., Winter, J. S., & Bressman, S. (2012). Toward a more effective mentoring model: An innovative program of collaboration. *Journal of Jewish Education, 78*(4), 331–361.	The study highlights three components of effective mentoring relationships: **Reflective dialogues:** Through reflective conversations mentors should encourage teachers to examine their classroom experiences, reflect on their successes, failures, and uncertainties, and assess newly gained experiential knowledge (Strong, 2009). **Basis of trust:** Effective mentoring relationships are built on foundations of trust and open communication (Levin & Rock, 2003; Yendol-Hoppey & Fitchman, 2007). Only when teachers sense a mentor's nonjudgmental role and commitment to confidentiality do they feel safe enough to share their puzzles, uncertainties, and concerns. **Meaningful Feedback:** Tension between two vital aspects of mentoring: trust and critical feedback. Enhancing teacher pedagogy while at the same time building a trusting and collaborative relationship. **Quotation:** "The affective nature of the social and emotional dimensions of the relationship with the teacher is essential for an effective and beneficial mentoring program" (p. 352).	Data collected from questionnaires given to the three groups involved in the program: teachers, mentors, and principals. Findings based only on open-ended surveys and on a limited number of participants. The tension between the mentor as assessor and as a confidant is also discussed in Hudson and Hudson.

GROUP WORK

1. Using your synthesis matrix, choose six articles to share with your group.
2. Read each other's analysis of the chosen articles as presented in the matrix.
3. Discuss the articles under each theme and subtheme using the following questions:
   a. Are the references listed according to APA or other chosen publication style rules?
   b. How clear and informative is the summary of each article? Will it be helpful in writing the literature review?
   c. Are the reflections useful in developing the next step of the literature review and are the critical responses logically presented?
   d. Do the articles under each theme enrich the understanding of the theme and illuminate its different aspects?
   e. How do the themes and subthemes relate to each other and how do the articles within each theme connect to each other?

SUMMARY TABLES

You can summarize the research studies that have a direct bearing on your topic in a single summary table. Such tables can help you organize the literature and assist in recalling and sorting information as you plan and write the review. In fact, a summary table can also be incorporated into your literature review narrative. Such a table helps the readers compare and contrast multiple studies in one glance. If there is too much information to be included in a single table, Pan (2013) suggests the use of one or more tables to summarize the literature. For example, you can create a table for summarizing qualitative or quantitative studies only, rather than including studies with different designs in a single table. You can also create several tables that focus on certain aspects of your subject, such as definitions, research methods, and findings.

HOW TO CONSTRUCT A SUMMARY TABLE

A comprehensive summary table like the template in Figure 7.1 (p. 130) allows you to organize and record your notes about a variety of research articles on your topic. In this table you can record: (1) the source where you found the article, (2) the purpose of the study, (3) the methodology used in the study, and (4) the major findings. The Sources column is further divided into three parts: Authors, Date, and Journal. Listing the references by their author(s) allows you to easily add, delete, and alphabetize sources, and including the date of publication provides information about the timeliness of the study. The Methodology column is divided into Design, Sample, and Data Collection Tools. This provides a quick reference to the design specifics of the study. Finally, the findings are summarized in a separate column. In this table, each research study is summarized in its own separate row.

Further information about each column is provided in the following sections. An example of a summary table follows the explanations.

Source				Methodology				
Author(s)	Date	Journal	Purpose	Design	Sample	Data collection tool(s)		Findings

FIGURE 7.1. Template of a summary table for research studies.

Source

The Source column is used to record information about the article and is divided into three columns. The first, Author, is designed to record the author(s) of the study, using the same format as you might use to refer to the author(s) in your review. Date of publication is listed next, followed by the title of the journal or other publication information that will help you obtain this article again if you wish to read it further or get additional information.

Purpose

The Purpose column is used to summarize the main goals and reasons for conducting the study, as presented by the authors. This information can often be found in the article's abstract or introduction.

Methodology

This column is further divided into three columns: Design, Sample, and Data Collection Tools. In the first column, record the design of the study (e.g., experimental, descriptive). For experimental studies, you may want to add information about the study's procedures and treatments. Information about the sample used in the study (e.g., the sample size and its demographic characteristics, and how it was selected) is included in the next column. Finally, a description of the tools that were used to collect data is included in the Data Collection Tools.

Findings

The last column is used to record the study's major findings. Following Galvan's (2013) advice, we recommend summarizing the findings in a narrative form rather than in statistical terms in order to more easily compare results from different studies and facilitate the interpretation of the findings.

You can develop your own abbreviation method. For example, you can use "J" instead of "Journal" or "Quant" and "Qual" to represent quantitative and qualitative design. You can also use other widely accepted shorthand notations such as N or n to denote a population or sample size, and "yrs" to represent "years."

An Example of a Summary Table

To illustrate how to use this summary table, let's look at the information gathered by Melinda, a doctoral student (whom we mentioned in Chapter 3) who is studying the topic of childhood depression and how to treat it. Her literature review yielded many studies on this important topic and she needed an efficient system to organize them. Figure 7.2 (pp. 132–135) shows excerpts from four of the studies Melinda analyzed and summarized for her review of the literature.

	Source			Methodology				
Author(s)	Date	Journal	Purpose	Design	Sample	Data collection tool(s)	Findings
Challen, Machin, & Gillham	2014	*Journal of Consulting & Clinical Psychology*, 82(1), 75–89	Assess the effectiveness of an 18-hr cognitive-behavioral group intervention in reducing depressive symptoms (and associated outcomes) in a universal sample of students in mainstream schools in England.	Quantitative; experimental; classes of students were assigned arbitrarily into intervention (UKRP) or control conditions based on class timetables; students surveyed at baseline, post intervention, 1-year follow-up, and 2-year follow-up.	N = 2,844; from 16 regions in the UK; 67% White, 49% female; ages 11–12; demographically varied, 25% eligible for free school lunch	Children's Depression Inventory; Revised Children's Manifest Anxiety Scale; Goodman Strengths and Difficulties Questionnaire	In post intervention, experimental group students reported lower levels of depressive symptoms than control group students, but the effect was small and did not persist to 1-year or 2-year follow-ups; no significant impact on symptoms of anxiety or behavior at any point. UKRP produced small, short-term impacts on depression symptoms and did not reduce anxiety or behavioral problems.
Garmy, Berg, & Clausson	2015	BMC Public Health,15, 1074	Explore adolescents' experiences with adolescent-based cognitive-behavioral depression prevention program	Qualitative assessment of intervention	N = 89; adolescents aged 13–15; divided into 12 focus groups designed to capture the experiences of adolescents who had participated in a school-based mental	Interviews were analyzed using qualitative content analysis. Transcripts were read repeatedly to achieve immersion and to obtain a sense of the whole picture. Sections of the text related to adolescents' experiences	Three categories and eight subcategories were found to be related to the experience of the school-based program. The first category, intrapersonal strategies, consisted of the subcategories of directed thinking, improved

(continued)

health program; the program consisted of 10 weekly manual-based sessions, each 90 minutes long with 7–18 students. The program is based on cognitive-behavioral techniques for changing negative thoughts, communication training, problem-solving strategies, exercises to strengthen social skills and social networks, and increased participation in health promotion activities.

participating in a school-based mental health program were combined into one text to form a content area. This text was divided into meaning units ($N = 478$), which were then condensed, abstracted, and labeled with codes. The context as a whole was considered during the condensing and coding process. The codes were compared on the basis of differences and similarities and sorted into three categories and eight subcategories. The first author conducted the first coding. The second and third authors independently coded two interviews each, and the three authors subsequently met and discussed the coding until they reached consensus. All authors reflected on and discussed the codes, categories, and subcategories throughout the analysis process to increase the level of trustworthiness.

self-confidence, stress management, and positive activities. The second category, interpersonal awareness, consisted of the subcategories of trusting the group and considering others. The third category, structural constraints, consisted of the subcategories of negative framing and emphasis on performance. Conclusions: The school-based mental health program was perceived as beneficial and meaningful on both individual and group levels, but students expressed a desire for a more health-promoting approach.

FIGURE 7.2. An excerpt from a summary table on the topic of treating childhood depression.

	Source				Methodology				Findings
Author(s)	Date	Journal	Purpose		Design	Sample	Data collection tool(s)		
McCann & Lubman	2012	*BMC Psychiatry, 12*(1), 96–104	Examine the experience of young people with depression accessing Australian Government recently established new enhanced primary care services (headspace) that target young people with emerging mental health issues with a focus on understanding how they access the service and the difficulties they encounter in the process.		Qualitative; descriptive	*N* = 26; in-depth, audio-recorded interviews were used to collect data. Participants with depression were recruited from a headspace site in Melbourne, Australia. Participants' ages ranged from 16–25, with a mean age of 18 years; 16 were young women, most were single; 15 lived in the same household as one or both parents; 6 were still attending high school; and 7 were engaged in various forms of paid employment; average length of engagement with the service was less than five months.	Purposive or criterion sampling was used to inform data collection. Inclusion criteria were: (i) primary diagnosis of depression, and (ii) aged 16–25 years. Exclusion criteria were (i) history of psychosis, (ii) currently expressing suicidal plans, and (iii) unable to communicate in conversational English. Interpretative phenomenological analysis was used to analyze the data. Interviews proceeded until no new themes were identified in the data. Furthermore, saturation of identified themes with "thick" description of the data was obtained when no new data emerged to support these themes. Each theme contained thick descriptions; deep, dense, depictions of the young people's experiences accessing the service. It was this process that determined the actual number of participants in the study (an important part of the rigor of the qualitative approach to determining sample size).		Four overlapping themes were identified in the data, reflecting the experiences of young people accessing the enhanced primary care service: (i) school counselors as service access mediators, (ii) service location as an access facilitator and inhibitor, (iii) encountering barriers accessing the service initially, and (iv) service funding as an access facilitator and barrier. Overall, the findings of this study indicate that while young people's experiences of accessing services share some similarities with adult consumers, such as the importance of establishing a trusting relationship with primary health care practitioners, there are important differences, including reliance on school counselors and use of informal access pathways; furthermore, because of the age of young people they are less likely to have the same social networks and help-seeking skills as adult consumers, which may delay their help-seeking efforts.

134

Author	Year	Source	Purpose	Design	Sample	Measures	Findings
Sifers & Mallela	2013	*Child and Adolescent Social Work Journal, 30,* 169–180	Examine relationship between hyperactivity and depression	Quantitative; descriptive	*N* = 100; 8- to 14-year-old students from public schools in a small Mid-western metropolitan area; equal gender ratio; 94% European-American; household; mean income of 79,949.	Social Support Scale for Children; Family Environment Scale; Behavioral Assessment System for Children, 2nd ed.	Hyperactivity is linked to difficulties in peer relationships, associated with depressive symptoms; hyperactivity is associated with a decrease in cohesion and an increase in conflict within the family, and with their levels of depressive symptoms. Relationship difficulties, both familial and nonfamilial, may be the conduit hrough which hyperactivity is linked to depressive symptoms.
Stice, Shaw, Bohon, Marti, & Rohde	2009	*Journal of Consulting and Clinical Psychology, 77*(3), 486–503		Quantitative; meta-analysis; descriptive	Authors identified 47 trials that evaluated 32 prevention programs, producing 60 intervention effect sizes; focus on trials that targeted children.	Five procedures were used to retrieve published and unpublished trials of depression prevention programs.	Among the 32 prevention programs that were evaluated in 60 trials, 13 produced significant reductions in depressive symptoms; 12 of the trials that produced significant effects found that intervention participants showed greater decreases in symptoms relative to decreases observed in controls, although one found that intervention participants showed a significant decrease in depressive symptoms, whereas controls showed a significant increase; intervention effects were significantly larger for high-risk participants, samples containing more females, and older adolescents.

FIGURE 7.2. *(continued)*

By using electronic data-recording tables, which you can create in Excel, you can organize your sources in a systematic way that will allow you to easily sort and retrieve information. For example, if you wish to further examine studies that were conducted using quantitative data, you can sort the table by the design column which will group together quantitative studies. Additionally, the use of an electronic table will allow you to write more detailed and specific notes or elaborate on certain points or on landmark studies, or on studies that are more directly related to your specific topic.

Our advice to you is to be creative and experiment with different formats of summary tables that will best meet your needs and help you organize and easily retrieve information!

GROUP WORK

1. Using your summary table, choose two articles to share with your group.

2. Read each other's analysis of the chosen articles as presented in the table.

3. Discuss the articles using the following questions:

   a. Are the sources listed in according with APA or other chosen publication style rules?

   b. Is the purpose of the study clearly explained and related to the literature review question(s)?

   c. Are there details provided about the study's methodology including its design, sample, and data collection tools?

   d. Are each article's findings summarized in a way that enables the comparison of results from different studies?

MAPPING THE LITERATURE

Mapping is a technique that uses a diagram to present the concepts and ideas included in the literature review. "Mapping out the ideas," claims Hart (1998), "is about setting out, on a paper, the geography of research and thinking that has been done on a topic" (p. 144). Organizing this "geography" visually helps the literature review writer recognize the connections and relationships among the research and theoretical conceptualizations and identify patterns that otherwise may be less apparent (Kalmer & Thomson, 2006). The pictorial presentation is useful for categorizing the different streams of research, identifying historical development of ideas, and noting schools of thought or other classifications (Daley & Torre, 2010). Such pictorial presentations may also be useful for illustrating to the reader the connections among the theoretical ideas and the research that are discussed in the literature review.

According to Hart (1998), mapping contributes to two kinds of literature knowledge: a declarative knowledge and a procedural knowledge. *Declarative knowledge* allows the writer to gain knowledge about theories, ideas, and concepts as presented in the literature. *Procedural knowledge* enhances the literature review author's ability to recognize how the above elements fit together and relate to one another. This, in turn, helps the writer review the literature written by others through his or her unique insight and understanding and then present it in a way that is original and creative.

There are different types of maps, among them mind maps, concept maps, topic flowcharts, cognitive maps, and flowcharts. Here we focus on two—the mind map and concept map—as examples of visual displays that will help you navigate and organize the information on your research topic.

The Mind Map

A mind map is a useful graphic device for organizing your thinking around individual major themes and defining their boundaries and subdivisions. The strength of this visual organization strategy lies in its simplicity (Ramanigopal, Palaniappan, & Mani, 2012). It is easy to construct and it does not require complex drawings or advanced graphic skills.

How to Construct a Mind Map

The list in Table 7.3 outlines the steps involved in constructing a mind map.

TABLE 7.3. Steps for Constructing a Mind Map
Step
1. Draw a circle and in its center write a main concept or theme from the literature.
2. Draw spoke lines leading from the circle outward.
3. Jot down at the end of each line the subtheme that is the subsidiary or supporting idea to the major theme in the circle.
4. Break down (when needed) the subthemes by extending spokes from them and recording additional narrower subconcepts.

While mind mapping can be easily performed without electronic methods, mapping software, such as FreeMind, LucidChart, MindMeister, and MindMup, may allow you to link the mind mapping with information you have summarized from the literature on each of the concepts.

Machi and McEvoy (2012) suggest using two kinds of mind maps for organizing the literature: mapping by core ideas and mapping by authors.

The Core Idea Map

The visual display of a *core idea map* assists you in centering your focus on individual major themes and organizing your analysis around different elements in the review relevant to these themes. These elements may be different theoretical positions, chronological development of ideas, or different definitions of a concept. ANTICs and thematic concentric circles (or even the synthesis matrix) may help you use keywords that will become a theme with its subthemes in your review. To illustrate the use of a core idea map, let's look at an example that Dave developed (see Figure 7.3). Dave, a doctoral student in counseling psychology, writes a paper about first-generation immigrants' level of success in their college studies. One of the major arguments in Dave's literature review is that one's identity is a key factor in the success of immigrant students. Dave uses a core idea map to reflect the different components that research claims contribute to identity formation.

The Author Map

The author map approach focuses on major figures related to your research topic. As you analyze the individual sources, you may recognize that the works of particular theoreticians or researchers are seminal in the development of the field and are central to your understanding of the topic. Constructing an author map may help you gain a deeper understanding of their positions as they relate to your own research or study. This map may also allow you to compare and contrast their ideas with the positions of other theoreticians or researchers.

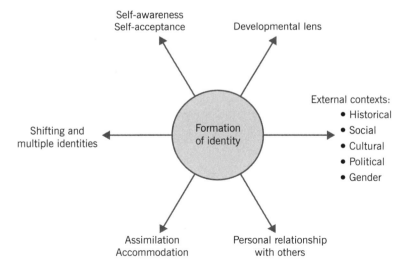

FIGURE 7.3. Core idea map: Identity formation. Based on Machi and McEvoy (2012).

As in any mind map, in an author map you extend a series of spokes from the circle at the center, in this case around the author's name. Drawing from his or her work, record the author's ideas and positions. For this map, you may use primary sources, as well as secondary sources in which the researcher's ideas and viewpoints are interpreted.

The use of an author map is illustrated by the way Rina, a sociology student, applied this approach to her research on democratic societies in the 20th century. In her reading, she was captivated by the idea developed by Hannah Arendt, a political theorist, about the role of dialogues with self and with others in forming a democratic citizen. Figure 7.4 shows an author map (based on Machi & McEvoy, 2012) that Rina developed while working on her literature review on Arendt's ideas.

As your work on the literature review progresses, we suggest developing iterative core idea maps or author maps for each of the major themes or central concepts that emerge as you read your sources. These maps can be modified and expanded as you continue reading the literature about these themes or authors.

Some writers like to develop mind maps concurrently with their work on the synthesis matrix. The matrix may serve as a helpful tool for identifying the concepts that will be at the center of their mind maps, and the core ideas or author

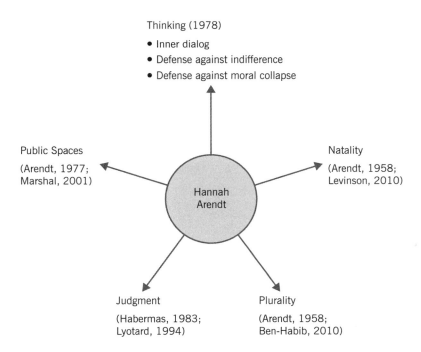

FIGURE 7.4. Author map: Hannah Arendt's concept of democracy.

maps will visually depict the subthemes within each theme and how they relate to each other.

The Concept Map

A concept map is a hierarchical structure that visually represents how different concepts are related to each other. The main difference between a mind map and a concept map is that the first is focused on a single concept while the latter reflects multiple concepts and the connections among them.

The advantage of a concept map is that it allows you to gain a holistic view of the literature review. The hierarchical diagram enhances your understanding of the general, as well as the specific, concepts within their overall context. In one glance, a full picture of the literature review components, their interconnections, and their structural organization unfolds before your eyes.

The concept map starts with broader concepts and through a hierarchical process narrows itself down to more specific ones. While there are many ways to construct the concept map, the process usually follows eight steps.

How to Construct a Concept Map

The list in Table 7.4 outlines the steps involved in constructing a concept map.

TABLE 7.4. Steps for Constructing a Concept Map
Step
1. Jot down a list of concepts that emerge from your readings. (You may be helped by your synthesis matrix.)
2. Write down, on the top of the page, the literature review's focus or question. (Most writers prefer using a landscape layout.)
3. Under the literature review focus write the broadest and most inclusive key concepts, from which all others stem.
4. From the list of concepts (see #1 above) identify those that branch out from the broadest concepts and record them underneath.
5. Continue downward in a progressively hierarchical pattern until the most specific concepts are listed.
6. Enclose the concepts in boxes, circles, or other geometric shapes.
7. Add lines to connect the concepts, possibly including a word or two to explain the relationships between them.

Some reviewers who use this organizing approach use different colors and various shapes as they construct their concept maps; others find this superfluous. Regardless of the style you choose, it is important that the concept map that you design is clear and that it concisely demonstrates the concepts and the relationships among them. Some researchers (e.g., Booth et al., 2008; Machi & McEvoy, 2012) suggest using Post-it index cards to construct the concept map and arranging them on a whiteboard or table horizontally and vertically according to ranking. They claim this enhances your flexibility and creativity in mapping the concepts by allowing you to move the cards around, add concepts, or change the relationships among them as you read additional articles.

A number of software programs have been developed to construct concept maps; among them are MindGenius, MindView, and SmartDraw. Alternatively, you may use traditional word-processing, presentation, and design programs such as Microsoft Word, Microsoft PowerPoint, Corel WordPerfect, or CorelDRAW to design different styles of concept maps. The advantage of the digital concept map programs is that they overcome the challenge of drawing clear and well-constructed concept maps by hand. Moreover, as your ideas evolve, using a digital map program makes it much easier to modify and revise your diagram.

Conversely, hand-drawn maps may enhance your thinking and stimulate your imagination. Advocates of hand-drawn concept maps feel that this approach allows them to come up with creative ideas they would not have not thought of before they actually started their design. Our suggestion is to be attuned to what works for you and follow that style.

An Example of a Concept Map

Figure 7.5 (p. 142) is an example of a concept map from a study conducted by Efron, Winter, and Bressman (2017) on the topic of mentoring across cultures. This concept map highlights the issues involved in this topic.

GROUP WORK

To assure the usefulness of the mind map and concept map you have constructed, share your outline with your group members and ask them to assess your map(s) using the checklist in Table 7.5 (p. 143).

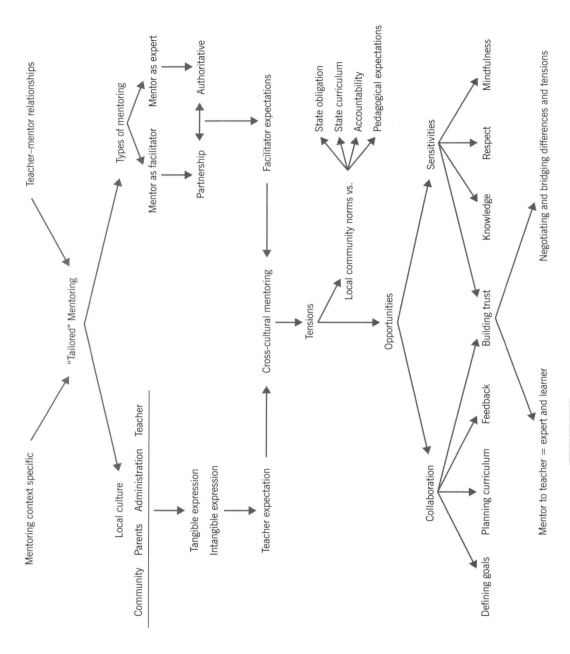

FIGURE 7.5. Concept map: Mentoring across cultures.

TABLE 7.5. A Checklist to Assess the Mind Map and/or Concept Map	
The mind map (theme/author) or concept map . . .	✓
1. Is developed in a way that responds purposefully to your research question.	
2. Includes concepts that reflect the central issues needed to understand the theme/author's ideas or the sources in the literature review.	
3. Offers a clear visual presentation of the concepts related to your research topic.	
4. Offers a clear and concise verbal presentation of the concepts related to your research topic.	
5. Demonstrates the relationships among the concepts or themes in the mind map.	
6. Offers a complete and inclusive list of the issues relevant to the theme/author or to your review.	
7. Has a hierarchical structure of the themes and subthemes that is logically constructed.	

OUTLINE

The last method you may want to consider for organizing the review of your sources is an outline. An outline is a structural plan that logically charts the main components of the literature review arranged in the order in which they will be discussed. It clearly distinguishes between major points and subordinate ones and guides the logical progression of the elements within the review (Wolcott, 2009). A well-constructed outline serves as a helpful blueprint for your literature review and makes the writing process easier and much more effective.

How to Construct an Outline

The list in Table 7.6 contains the steps involved in constructing an outline.

TABLE 7.6. Steps for Constructing an Outline
Step
1. Revisit the notes you have written for each reference in the Article Note-Taking Index Cards (ANTICs) and group them together according to their common focus in order to identify the major themes of your outline. The key terms you used to label your summaries will help you in this effort. (If you already have created the synthesis matrix or mind maps, this phase will be much faster and easier.)
2. Check the ANTICs again and select issues that fall logically under the major themes and can serve as subthemes. These subdivisions represent more specific information that defines, explains, or supports facets of the major themes.
3. If the subthemes are still too broad, divide them into narrower categories.

The selection of the themes, subthemes, and categories in your outline is based on your research purpose and the questions that undergird your review, as well as the references included in your review. Constructing an outline provides you with an opportunity to revisit your questions and see whether, after the readings that you have done, they still reflect your research focus or need to be revised.

As you develop the outline, you have to make three choices. The first one relates to the *format* of the outline, the second to the *style* of the outline, and the third to the way you *order* the themes and subthemes in your outline.

Outline Format

The basic format for the outline uses a series of numbers and letters according to their level of importance. The letters or numbers at each level are aligned at the same indentation and are structured as following:

1. The **first** level of the outline, the major themes, is labeled with uppercase Roman numerals: **I, II, III**, etc.

2. The **second** level of the outline, the subthemes, is indented and labeled with uppercase letters: **A, B, C**, etc.

3. The **third** level of the outline, the categories, is indented again and labeled with Arabic numerals: **1, 2, 3**, etc.

4. The **fourth** level of the outline is indented again and labeled with lowercase letters: **a, b, c**, etc.

5. If additional subcategories are needed, indent again and use lowercase Roman numerals: i, ii, iii, etc.

According to the rules, there can't be a single item in a subset. There have to be at least two entries.

The outline format may look like this:

I. _____

   A. _____

   B. _____

      1. _____

      2. _____

         a. _____

         b. _____

            i. _____

            ii. _____

Some writers (e.g., Booth et al., 2008; Wolcott, 2009) view this formalistic approach with its emphasis on indenting, numbering, and rigid rules as too complex and limiting. While they recognize the advantages of an outline, they prefer a simpler, more loosely structured format that allows the imagination to flow without the "nuisance" of keeping all the above rules in mind.

Outline Style

Your second decision in developing the outline is choice of style. There are two common choices:

▶ A topic outline that consists of very few words or short phrases

▶ A sentence outline that uses full sentences

Booth at al. (2008) suggest that each of these styles of outlines can be useful at different stages in the development of the literature review. At earlier stages of writing, when you just start to construct your ideas and concepts, you may prefer using a topic outline. However, at a later stage, as you continue reading and analyzing articles and other sources, a sentence outline is more useful. Such an outline helps you see whether your ideas hang together and flow logically one from another. Additionally, topic outlines lack clear specificity, and after a while, when you revisit your topic outline, it may seem too vague and you may not recall the exact meaning of your short phrases. A full-sentence outline, on the other hand, may trigger your memory and remind you of the ideas you had when writing the topic outline's entries. Some writers prefer to combine the two styles and use complete sentences for the major topics and short phrases for the subtopics and narrower categories.

An Example of an Outline

The following is an example of an outline based on the literature review chapter in Dr. Barbara Sherman's (2014) dissertation that was described above.

BOX 7.1. Scholarship Students: Squeezing through the Glass Ceiling of an Affluent Private School

I. Introduction to field of study

   A. The importance of understanding the historical, social, political, and educational contexts that impact scholarship students

   B. Major issues discussed in the literature review

(continued)

BOX 7.1. *(continued)*

II. Early immigrants to America (late 18th–early 20th century)

   A. Creating social hierarchy as waves of immigrants face cultural norms (Ramirez et al., 2008)

   B. Racism-serving scientific theory

      1. Using "scientific" means to classify immigrants into racial categories (Jackson & Weidman, 2006)

      2. Social Darwinism: connecting race to abilities and survival potential (Darwin, 1871; Jeynes, 2011; Spencer, 1851)

      3. Eugenics movement's Immigration Restriction League (Immigration Restriction League's web page, Harvard University)

   C. Prejudice, racism, and discrimination are socially constructed

      1. Defining the concepts of prejudice, racism and discrimination (Katz, 1978)

      2. Political, economic, and social circumstances' impact on perception of the social other (Higham, 1983; Perry, 2010)

      3. Attitude toward the Asian immigrant (Tan, 1989), the South American immigrant (Rosenblum. Soelke, & Wasem, 2012) and the African American (Ogbu, 1978; Tim, 1992)

III. Educational response to the surge of immigrants

   A. Keeping the "other" outside the mainstream or assimilating them? (Zangwill, 1976)

      1. Espoused principles of equality vs. realities of discrimination (De Hoyus, 2012; Ramsey & Williams, 2003)

      2. Educate immigrants and encourage their assimilation into "American culture" (Ramsey & Williams, 2003)

      3. American Indians join the melting pot to become "true Americans" (Manuelo, 2005)

   B. Segregation of community and of school

      1. Laws to ensure segregation: Jim Crow and *Plessey v. Ferguson* of 1896 (Wright, 2009)

      2. Horace Mann's Common School vs. segregation (Cayton et al., 2003)

      3. The story of Malcolm Little (Malcolm X) as a story of discrimination against African American children (Haley, 1999)

   C. Cultural pluralism: Marginal communities fight to retain their culture

      1. 1920s curriculum programs supportive of cultural pluralism and embracing immigration (Ratner, 1984)

      2. Black leaders of the 1940s make demands for equal opportunity in employment, schooling, and the armed forces (De Hoyos, 2013)

      3. The Black Power movement demands equal rights (De Hoyos, 2013)

      4. Rising of Latino and Asians movements (Brown Power and Yellow Power)

(continued)

BOX 7.1. *(continued)*

IV. Turning point: American education begins to embrace diversity

   A. Attempts to Create Equality between the Races (Norton, 2002)

      1. The effects of *Brown vs. Board of Education* on schools (Patterson, 2001)

      2. Hilda Taba's Intergroup Education Movement (Banks, 2007; Norton, 2002)

      3. Education and the Civil Right Movement: 1960 (Cayton, 2003; Patterson, 2001)

      4. Reform of the immigration policy: New Immigration Policy (1965) (Ludden, 2006)

   B. Education supports multiculturalism: 1970s

      1. Cultural pluralism evolves into multicultural education (Banks, 2001; Ramsey & Williams, 2003)

      2. Goals of multicultural education (Grant, 1978)

      3. Multicultural education adopts social deconstructionism (Nieto, 2012)

      4. White race identity theory (Helms, 1990)

V. The achievement gap

   A. Disparity in achievement between races (Ladson-Billings, 2009; NAEP, 2009)

      1. Role of class and economics in the achievement gap (Scott & Lonhardt, 2009)

      2. Narrowing the achievement gap (National Assessment of Education Progress, 2009; The Quiet Revolution: Secretary Arne Duncan's Remarks at the National Press Club, 2010)

      3. Cultural vs. sociopolitical roots of the achievement gap (Hilliand, 1992; Ladson-Billing, 2001, 2009; Ogbu, 1999; Williams, 1996)

VI. Telling only one story endangers curriculum

   A. Marginalizing a group by a single image (Adichie, 2009)

      1. The power of the written word in creating and destroying images of groups of people (Horn, 2003; Katz & Earp (1999)

      2. Media image of minority youth (Katz & Earp, 1999)

   B. The message of hidden curriculum (Audre Lorde, as cited in Tatum, 1997, p. 22)

      1. Defining hidden curriculum (Giroux & Penna, 1979; Murrell, 2007)

      2. Hidden curriculum creates barriers (Grunty, 1987; Jardine, 2006; Langhout, 2008)

         a. Two approaches to hidden curriculum: The functionalist approach and the neo-Marxist approach (Anyon, 1980; Apple, 1980; Lynch, 1989)

         b. Hidden agenda determined by hegemony (Sari & Doganay, 2009)

(continued)

BOX 7.1. *(continued)*

    3. Institutional discrimination: A product of hidden curriculum (Anyon, 1980; Freire, 1970; Murrell, 2007)

        a. Cultural Capital (Bourdieu, 1986; Yosso, 2005)

        b. School as political institution (Dewey, 1916; Freire, 1970)

    4. Hidden curriculum's impact on human dignity (Sari & Doganay, 2009)

    5. Hidden curriculum's reinforcement of social constructs (Anyon, 1980; Tyack, 1993)

VII. Challenges of pursuing an education in private schools

    A. From poorly resourced schools to affluent private schools (Murell, 2007)

        1. Definition of cultural competence (Ingram, 2011)

        2. The role of cultural competence in successful integration (Banks, 1981, 1987)

    B. Stigmatizing students without cultural competencies (Salzman, 2005)

        1. Knowledge deemed worth knowing (Bullhan, 1985; Pinar et al., 2008)

        2. Deficit theory and its consequences (Hale, 2011)

    C. The impact of race on social relationships within schools (Baldwin, 1971; Castnell & Pinar, 1993; Fanon, 1970; Pinar, 2008)

VIII. School responsibility: Creating democratic citizens in practice

    A. School's role in a democratic society (Dewey, 1916, 1959; Horn, 2003; Pinar, 2008)

        1. Human dignity as the root of democratic values (Kaboglu, 2002)

        2. Practicing democracy in school community (Jardine et al., 2006; Sari & Doganay, 2009)

    B. Unpacking the "Monster" in the curriculum (Nall, 1999)

        1. Curriculum conflicts with the teaching of democracy (Dewey, 1959)

        2. Culturally sensitive teaching (Banks & Banks, 1995; Gay, 2000)

        3. Diversity in schools enriches education (Troyna & Hatch, 1992)

IX. Diversity in schools enriches education (summary and discussion)

GROUP WORK

To assure the usefulness of the outline you have constructed, share it with your group members and ask them to assess it using the checklist in Table 7.7.

TABLE 7.7. A Checklist to Assess the Outline	
The Outline . . .	✓
1. Is developed in a way that responds purposefully to your research question.	
2. Offers a holistic presentation of the state of knowledge related to your research topic.	
3. Is properly sequenced and flows logically from one idea to the next.	
4. Is complete and inclusive of all the issues relevant to your review.	
5. Does not include repetitive or irrelevant items that stall the progress of your review.	
6. Does not have entries that should be combined or divided.	
7. Includes different or even contradictory opinions or perceptions.	
8. Has entries that are clearly and concisely stated.	
9. Is not too detailed or too brief.	
10. Cites the authors and publication dates of the sources used in the entries.	

Outline Organization

The third decision, and probably the most important one you make as you develop your outline, is how to organize it. Your decision should be based on your purpose in writing the review and the literature you included. There is no one single way in which the outline should be organized; rather, you have the freedom to choose how to structure it. With the exception of preparing an outline for a systematic review (that is further discussed below), you may structure the review in a way that you deem fit as long as the themes are progressing logically and there is a coherent and purposeful movement from one idea to the next.

In the following section we describe some of the most common organizational approaches: thematic outline, chronological outline, outline separating the theoretical from the empirical, theoretical to methodological outline, systematic review outline, and hermeneutic–phenomenological review outline. Examples are provided to illustrate the distinguishing characteristics of each approach. These examples represent the major topics of the review and do not include the subtopics.

Thematic

The most commonly used approach to outline organization is based on dividing it into themes. The distinct themes around which the entries are organized may surface from the literature or may be predetermined. Each theme may integrate both theoretical writings and empirical studies that are related to the research topic. Box 7.2 presents an example of a thematic outline on the topic of assessment developed by Joseph for his master's thesis in educational leadership.

Chronological

An outline may be organized chronologically with the major topics ordered around time periods. This organizational approach is uniquely suitable for subjects that have changed over time. The entries in the outline indicate the major time periods (from earlier dates to the present) that mark the historical developments of the subject. A review based on such organization may explore chronologically the progress of theories, emergence of policies, development of research methods, or changes in practices. This organizational approach allows the writer to discern changing trends over time. An example of such organization (Box 7.3, p. 151) was chosen by Mina for a research paper about the historical cycles of reform in education from the post–World War II period to the present.

Separation of the Theoretical from the Empirical

If you have identified multiple sources, both theoretical and empirical, you may want to divide the review into two distinct sections. In the first part, your review can focus on theoretical and conceptual studies, while in the second part your attention will center on empirical studies (quantitative and/or qualitative), their methodologies, and their findings. Some researchers (e.g., Carnwell & Daly, 2001; Ridley, 2012) assert that if you have chosen this type of review, you should not be satisfied with merely describing the literature, but rather adopt a critical stance.

BOX 7.2. An Example of Thematic Outline Organization

   I. Different perceptions of assessment in history
  II. Summative assessment (theories, research, and practice)
 III. Formative assessment (theories, research, and practice)
 IV. Assessment by systems
  V. Assessment by teachers
 VI. Assessment by students

BOX 7.3. An Example of Chronological Outline Organization

    I. Cold War in school—The impact of Russia launching Sputnik (1957)

    II. The Civil Rights Movement—Elementary and Secondary Education Act (1967)

    III. Nation at Risk—Expanding the federal role (1983)

    IV. No Child Left Behind—The children who were left behind (2002)

    V. Common Core: Opportunities, challenges, risks (2010s)

    VI. Reforming No Child Left Behind—Every Student Succeeds Act (2015)

    VII. Reflections: The expanding role of government in enforcing accountability and standardization.

An example of this kind of organization can be found in Box 7.4. It is an outline of a review written by Magda, who trains counselors and is now getting ready to defend her doctoral dissertation. The focus of her research is the development of cultural competency among counselors-in-training.

Theoretical to Methodological

When the sources you have found in the literature on your topic are mostly theoretical and you have located very few or no empirical references, you may consider this type of organization, which is divided into two parts. The first part is a theoretical discussion on conceptual frameworks and the schools of thought underpinning your subject and the differences and commonalities among them. The second part consists of an exploration of a research approach that complements the identified theories discussed in the first part and may lead to your research question. An

---

BOX 7.4. An Example of Separation-of-the-Theoretical-from-the-Empirical Outline Organization

    I. Defining culture and its role in relationships

    II. Multicultural competency theory

    III. The implications of multicultural competency theory for the counseling field

    IV. Self-awareness among novice counselors-in-training of the role of multicultural competency in counseling

    V. Critical analysis of the methods currently practiced to develop multicultural competency in counseling programs

    VI. Research-based recommendations for developing multicultural competencies for counselors

BOX 7.5. An Example of Theoretical-to-Methodological Outline Organization

   I. Feminism and cultural hegemony

  II. Evolution of thought toward feminist theory

 III. Transnational feminist theory

 IV. Summary of thoughts

  V. The power of stories that matter: A feminist perspective

 VI. Narrative as a research design

example of this type of an organization is the outline in Box 7.5 based on April's dissertation in sociology, whose literature review focused on transnational feminine theory.

Systematic Review

This approach is specifically intended for writers of systematic reviews. This type of review does not allow writers flexibility nor freedom in developing the organization of their literature review, but rather expects them to strictly follow a required discussion structure (Booth et al., 2016). In order to enhance the researcher's ability to systematically compare studies on the basis of variables, such as sample characteristics, research design, or results, the systematic review approach dictates how the outline should be constructed. A typical structure of such a review can be found in Box 7.6.

BOX 7.6. An Example of Systematic Review Outline Organization

   I. Formulating the research question

  II. Criteria for including studies

 III. Methods for searching the literature

 IV. Data extraction (examines which elements of data are presented in each study)

  V. Data analysis (evaluates and summarizes studies in a table format)

 VI. Results and interpretation

VII. Discussion and implications

Hermeneutic–Phenomenological

The last approach to literature review organization is appropriate for hermeneutic–phenomenological inquiries (Boell & Cecez-Kemanovic, 2014). In structuring an outline for this type of review, a particular framework is used to present the discourse on a chosen topic. An example of such a structure can be seen in a chapter of James Magrini's dissertation (2014). In this chapter, Magrini's discussion of the work of van Manen and Heidegger in relation to selfhood leads him to criticize the current accountability and standardization trends in education. Using the hermeneutic–phenomenological lenses, he identifies gaps, reveals weaknesses, and problematizes the dominant language that typifies current educational research and practice. This hermeneutic–phenomenological approach to outline organization can be found in Box 7.7.

BOX 7.7. An Example of Hermeneutic–Phenomenological Outline Organization

  I. The unfolding of hermeneutic–phenomenological interpretation

  II. Positivism and losing or forgetting of phenomenological and ontological selfhood

  III. Critique of the language of standardized learning

  IV. Learning as understood in phenomenological-ontological terms.

FINAL COMMENTS

As you plan the organization of your review, experiment with different ways of ordering your themes. Developing an outline is an iterative process and you do not want to be locked into a single form before you are ready to write your review. As you continue reading and analyzing your sources, don't be controlled by the themes or subthemes you have identified. Whenever you note something in a source that supports, explains, or contradicts, add it to your existing themes or construct a new one. Every now and then, check whether your organization of the review is still suitable or if a new order is needed. Remember, an outline is a living organism (Dawidowicz, 2010) that requires an openness to revisions.

Additionally, whatever outline organizational strategy you choose for structuring your review, keep in mind that in the end the literature review—unless it is a stand-alone review—should lead smoothly and logically to your own research. Consider the process as a funnel, where the discussion about the topic starts from a wide angle that eventually and gradually narrows to focus on your own research question. Therefore, as you come closer to the end of the review you should zoom in on studies that are most similar or most relevant to your own particular research (Wellington et al., 2005).

In this chapter we offered several strategies for logically organizing the information you have obtained through the analysis of the individual sources you have deemed as relevant to your literature review. These strategies are: synthesis matrix, summary table, mind map and concept map, and topical outline. Each of the strategies may serve to identify patterns, highlight themes, and note relationships that will allow you to build a logical flow and reveal your review's story line. Having a choice between several kinds of strategies enables you to select the ones that best suit your learning style, serve your particular goals in writing the review, and reflect the nature of your review.

Play with the different strategies until you feel that you found those that will enhance your writing. You may want to alternate among the strategies, combine several of them, or develop you own distinct way of classifying and organizing your literature review. This is an imaginative, innovative, and purposeful process that will allow you to assemble the building blocks to reveal the whole picture.

GROUP WORK

In this chapter we discussed several organizational styles: synthesis matrix, summary table, mind map and concept map, as well as an outline. In your group, consider which one or more of these organizational strategies will be useful for your literature review writing. This decision can be based on your purpose in writing the review, the literature included, and your self-awareness of your personal learning style.

In your group discussion, each of you should respond to the following questions:

1. Will you use one or more of the organizational strategies offered in this chapter? Explain why.

2. How does your chosen organizational strategy reflect the purpose of your literature review and the articles you will include in your writing? Explain.

3. Explain how your chosen organizational strategy reflects your personal learning style.

WHAT'S NEXT?

In this chapter we described the strategies most often used for organizing the literature review; these strategies offer different ways to logically construct your narrative. The following chapter focuses on constructing your literature review arguments.

CHAPTER SUMMARY

1. Methods used by researchers to construct their literature review differ from each other in their organization techniques, formats of presentation, and the types of structure that they highlight.

2. The *synthesis matrix* enables researchers to achieve an overview of the literature, providing a succinct organization of the tentative and iterative topical themes and subthemes of the narrative.

3. A *summary table* is used to sum up research studies that have a direct bearing on the topic. Such tables help to organize, retrieve, and easily sort information about the different studies.

4. There are different formats for summary tables, among them *mapping, mind map, core idea map,* and *author map*.

5. A *concept map* is a hierarchical structure that visually represents how different concepts are related to each other. It starts with broader concepts and through a hierarchical process narrows itself down to more specific ones.

6. A *topic outline* is a structural plan that logically charts the main components of the literature review, arranged in the order in which they will be discussed.

7. The selection of the themes, subthemes, and categories in the topic outline is based on the research purpose and the questions that undergird the review, as well as the references that are included in the review.

8. As you develop the topic outline, there are three choices to be made. The first one relates to the *format* of the outline, the second to the *style* of the outline, and the third to the *order* of the themes and subthemes.

9. Common organizations of an outline are: thematic, chronological, separating the theoretical from the empirical, theoretical to methodological, systematic review, and hermeneutic–phenomenological review.

10. Developing an outline is an iterative process, and as you continue reading and analyzing your sources, don't be controlled by the outline you have developed.

Developing Arguments and Supporting Claims

A t its core, the literature review is centered on the question(s) you have formulated in regard to your research topic and on building a case for your own research study. You may address both of these issues by putting forward an argument that focuses on your topic of interest and leads to your own research. This argument should draw from and build upon the texts you have read on your subject. As you construct your literature review, you analyze, synthesize, and critique multiple pieces of research, weave them together, and lay brick by brick the claims that build your argument. This argument should not merely echo the ideas of authors whose writings you have reviewed, but rather advance or expand what is known and present it from your own unique perspective. Your construction of the current state of knowledge "involves some degree of conceptual innovation" (Strike & Posner, 1983, p. 52) and demonstrates that while you are deeply familiar with the up-to-date scholarship in your field, you are not controlled by it (Ridley, 2012).

In the previous chapters, we discussed the creative process of data extraction and critical analysis of individual sources in order to identify key terms and emerging themes. We suggested grouping studies around these themes and developing a visual display or an outline that organizes and depicts the relationships among them. This process of organization and visualization provides a degree of clarity and coherence that allows you to put together a sound argument. While the steps we described seem like a linear course of actions, argument building, like any phase in the literature development, is a recursive procedure. This process is tentative, continually evolving, and requires the writer to move back to earlier stages of the literature review development as well as make leaps ahead (Douglas, 2014). Thus, you do not need to wait to build your argument until you have read all your references. Rather, at an earlier stage, you may (perhaps tentatively) decide what argument will drive your literature review (Booth et al., 2008).

An argument in the context of literature review writing is your main idea, a position that you put forward to reflect your standpoint on the topic. Without having such an argument your literature review faces the hazard of being a mere information dump where studies, concepts, and theories are piled up one upon the other in a muddled display. Your argument, which is supported by evidence, is presented in order to persuade your audience that what you propose is justified (Booth et al., 2008; Hart, 1998; Jesson et al., 2011; Machi & McEvoy, 2012; Ridley, 2012).

According to Machi and McEvoy (2012), in most literature reviews there are two kinds of basic arguments and they name them *argument of discovery* and *argument of advocacy*. Argument of discovery presents what is known about the subject at the center of your research; whereas the argument of advocacy focuses on the meaning of this knowledge and how to expand and extend it. These two kinds of arguments differ in their goals and in the way they are constructed.

This chapter contains two parts: the first focuses on building an argument of discovery. We focus first on constructing a simple argument that consists of three basic elements: claim, evidence, warrant. We then describe four patterns of argument that differ from each other in their level of complexity: one-on-one reasoning, independent reasoning, dependent reasoning, and chain reasoning. The second part is focused on argument of advocacy. We discuss how to conclude the literature review by interpreting the meaning of what was learned through the literature in the context of your own intended study or future action.

BUILDING AN ARGUMENT

A literature review's argument may come in various patterns backed by different types of evidence. There are, however, basic rules for constructing arguments. To understand these rules, our discussion focuses first on constructing a simple argument before we illustrate how an argumentation may become more intricate and complex.

Simple Argument

A simple argument consist of three basic elements, the claim, the evidence, and the warrant (Booth et al., 2008; Hart, 1998; Machi & McEvoy, 2012).

▶ **Claim:** An assertion, a statement, an idea that is being argued.
▶ **Evidence:** Data gathered to support the claim.

▶ **Warrant:** A bridge that connects evidence to claim and explains how the data support that claim.

Booth et al. (2008) explain that every argument is formed by answering the following questions:

1. What is your claim?
2. What evidence justifies your support of the claim?
3. What is the underlying assumption that connects the evidence to your claim?

Box 8.1 illustrates how those elements are used. This example is based on the dissertation of Karen, a public high school teacher and coach, who began her literature review discussion by expressing her concerns about teacher attrition.

As you construct a claim, you should consider two aspects: the *type* of claim and the *quality* of claim.

Type of Claims

Hart (1998) suggests five primary types of claims that are most often used in literature review: Claims of fact, worth, policy, concept, and interpretation. To illustrate what distinguishes each type of claim, we are using the topic of youth incarceration:

▶ *Claim of fact.* The writer proposes something as a settled fact or truth. An example for such a claim is the following: "Minority youth are being incarcerated in public juvenile correctional facilities at rates three times higher than white youth."

BOX 8.1. An Example of the Use of Claim, Evidence, and Warrant

Claim: Administrators are worried about the high attrition rate among new teachers.

Evidence: About one-third of all beginning teachers leave the profession within the first 3 years, and approximately 50% of teachers leave the field by the end of the fifth year (Ingersoll, Merrill, & May, 2014).

Warrant: A high level of novice teacher turnover presents a severe challenge for the educational system.

▶ *Claim of value.* The writer asserts the merit of theory, idea, phenomenon, or course of action and declares whether it is good or bad, desirable or not. An example of such a claim is the following: "Incarceration of adolescents has destructive implications for their emotional, psychological, and social development."

▶ *Claim of policy.* The writer argues that one course of action is preferable in comparison to another. An example of such a claim is the following: "To reduce the level of incarceration of adolescents, the community should implement effective interventions rather than using the punitive measure of juvenile correctional facilities"

▶ *Claim of concept.* The writer presents a definition of a concept or a description of a phenomenon. An example of such a claim is the following: "*School-to-prison-pipeline* refers to the punitive journey taken by minority youth from public school to juvenile justice system."

▶ *Claim of interpretation.* The writer provides a statement that offers a framework for understanding data or evidence. An example of such a claim is the following: "Based on the findings we can assert that students' grade retention during the high school years increases the likelihood of their dropping out of formal education, which in turn may lead to higher rates of incarceration."

Which types of claim are right for your particular review will depend on your overall argument and the context of your work. You will probably utilize several of these types of claims in your narrative. Regardless of the type of claim you are using, all of them must be supported by evidence.

Quality of Claim

The claims present the position that drives your argument. You want to be sure that your argument persuades your audience to accept the trustworthiness of your claim and see it as convincing and justified. To achieve that goal, the claim should be on point, precise, and significant (Booth et al., 2008). This means the following:

▶ *On point.* Claims should be valid, directly related to the argument you put forward, and strengthen its soundness.

▶ *Precise.* Vague claims lead to a vague argument. Vagueness may be due to a lack of clear definition or to a mistaken use of concepts. The more specific, accurate, and clearly stated your language is, the better understood and more convincing your argument will be.

▶ *Significant.* The claim should not be trivial or meaningless. It should provide a strong basis for your argument and subsequently lead to addressing your review question.

Do not stop with just proposing a claim; in a literature review, claims have to be backed up with evidence. The soundness of your claim also depends on the quality of the evidence you offer.

Evidence

Evidence is data that is used to back up a claim. However, there is a difference between data and evidence (Machi & McEvoy, 2012). Whereas data are made of value-free information, evidence is data presented to establish the validity of the claim you argue. In your literature review you need to provide data that will be used as evidence to justify your claims and viewpoints. Personal opinions, beliefs, and positions that are not accompanied by evidence will not contribute to your ability to make a persuasive argument. Some fields of study allow literature review writers to respond to claims drawn from the literature by sharing anecdotal experiences and personal beliefs and insights. However, these personal and experiential opinions can never, on their own, serve as a ground for a sound claim (Machi & McEvoy, 2012). The evidence for the claim you present should come from empirical (quantitative or qualitative) data, as well as from conceptual, theoretical, or philosophical works written by scholars in your field or in related areas.

The credibility of a claim relies on the quality of the evidence you use to support it and the evidence's strength depends on the data you present. It is important that you use the right kind of data and that it is used effectively; it has to be accurate, precise, authoritative, representative, current, and relevant (Booth et al., 2008; Machi & McEvoy, 2012). This means the following:

▶ *Accurate.* The quantitative evidence must be based on sound methods, represented in a consistent and unambiguous form, and devoid of systematic errors and biases. When it comes to qualitative data, there should be a detailed description of the participants, settings, and participants' points of view, as well as the researcher's subjectivity.

▶ *Precise.* When describing statistical data, state the evidence precisely, including, when appropriate, the exact statistical probability. Avoid terms such as *mostly, some, often,* and *usually* and consider the population to which the evidence can be reasonably applied. For qualitative data, the research process and procedures used during the inquiry should be described in detail and consideration should be given to the social and cultural context of the evidence.

▶ *Authoritative.* Data are trusted when the findings cited as evidence are based on studies whose procedures are appropriate for the questions asked and are adequately implemented. When it comes to using theories and philosophical sources, the evidence draws from the writings of credible scholars in or in related fields.

▶ *Representative.* The data represent populations that match those at the center of your research. Be sure that no particular group among them is overrepresented, underrepresented, or misrepresented. When outliers are used in qualitative studies, their use is clearly stated and explained. Additionally, the evidence you present should reflect different approaches and be obtained through different methods.

▶ *Current.* The evidence that supports claims, especially when drawing on empirical studies, should mostly be based on current research. Although citations of classical theoreticians or the use of past research is valuable when presenting a historical perspective, cite current research to justify your argument.

▶ *Relevant.* The data you present as evidence should be directly related to the claim. The studies cited should reflect the specifics of your study in terms such as *population, social context,* and *treatment.*

The purpose of the evidence is to substantiate the claim. Thus, there should be a clear, logical link between the evidence and the claim it is supposed to support. Without that link, even if the evidence is credible and valid, the review reader may not accept the conclusions proposed by the claim. To ensure this purposeful link, the third element of argument, the warrant, is used.

Warrant

The third element of an argument is a warrant. The warrant is a provision or a logical principle that supports the claim by using a sound link that justifies the connection between the evidence and the claim (Booth et al., 2008; Hart, 1998). It offers a general principle of reasoning that serves as a basic premise from which the writer makes the claim and presents the evidence as a plausible instance of the generalization. There are warrants that are explicitly *stated* and those that are *unstated* but are implicitly implied in the claim.

An example of a stated warrant is taken from Paul Reiff's (2016) dissertation on the importance of aesthetics in school curriculum. In Reiff's example (Box 8.2, p. 162), the warrant highlights the contributions of aesthetic experience in general. This warrant serves as a link between the claim that argues for the need to integrate the arts into schools, and the evidence of the impact of aesthetic education on students' development drawn from curriculum thinkers' writings.

To assure that the warrant strengthens the persuasiveness of the argument, the writer needs to ensure that:

1. The assumption embedded within the general principle is widely regarded as valued among the author's audience.

2. The logic behind the warrant clearly applies to both the specific claim and the particular evidence that are put forward.

BOX 8.2. An Example of a Stated Warrant

Warrant

The power of aesthetic experience lies in its ability to put us in touch with some-thing transcendent and universal that moves us to aspire and to strive upward, beyond ourselves.

Claim

Aesthetic experiences should be integral to schools' curriculum rather than being shunned.

Evidence

Greene (2001) describes aesthetic education as a process of initiating students into "faithful perceiving" (p. 45), a means of empowering them to come to their own unique understandings accomplished from their own standpoints and against the background of their own individual awareness. . . . Schools are morally obligated to attend to these kinds of values, Greene concludes.

Source: Based on Reiff's (2016) doctoral dissertation.

As stated above, there are also claims that do not include stated warrants. There are many reasons for using unstated warrants; most of them derive from one of two factors: (1) the author feels that the backing evidence's reason is clearly linked to the claim and there is no need for a connecting principle or (2) the writer assumes that the readers are familiar with the assumption underlying the claim and stating it is redundant. Box 8.3 is an example of an argument without a warrant, although the generalized principle is embedded within the claim and its evidence.

The unstated warrants underlying the claim in Box 8.3 might be (1) standardized test scores are an accurate measurement tool for evaluating students' academic performance or (2) student academic gains are not influenced by socioeconomic background, limited English, or learning or behavior challenges. The writer assumes that the reader accepts these two points although this may not be the case.

BOX 8.3. An Example of a Claim with Unstated Warrants

Any educational system should link the assessment of teacher quality to their students' academic achievement. Research employing longitudinal data has shown that teachers' effectiveness is a major factor influencing students' gain in standardized test scores (Borman & Kimball, 2005; Fong-Yee, 2013; Goe & Stickler, 2008).

In addition to the three elements included in an argument, claim, evidence, and warrant, there are three more components that are important for establishing the soundness of a claim: qualifier, backing, and counter claim (Booth et al., 2008; Hart, 1998; Machi & McEvoy, 2012; Toulmin, 2003).

Qualifier

In their efforts to persuade readers of the strength of their argument some novice literature review writers inflate their claims by asserting their universality (i.e., something is always and everywhere true). However, predictions in social and human sciences, as well as in education, are generally subject to changing conditions; therefore, claims stated in these disciplines often have exceptions or limitations.

To make your argument more credible, it should consist of a qualifier that proposes the conditions under which the claim is true (Booth et al., 2008; Toulmin, 2003). For example, the following claim is too overreaching:

> The social capital theory proposes that the trust, reciprocity, information, and collaboration associated with social networks benefit *all the people* who are connected to these networks.

More appropriate and probably closer to reality is narrowing and stating the claim as follows:

> The social capital theory proposes that the trust, reciprocity, information, and collaboration associated with social networks benefit *most of the people* who are connected to these networks.

You narrow the claim by either reducing its scope (e.g., demographics, age, gender, ethnic background, and location) or by limiting the condition of the claim: "If done during . . . ," "If implemented according to . . . ," "If all participants share the conceptual idea behind. . . ." Words such as *most, some, many, majority, generally, usually,* and *often* are frequently used by authors to qualify their conclusions and indicate their recognition that their claims are not absolute and have some limitations (Toulmin, 2003).

Backing

Many arguments may also include definitions or background information needed to understand the meaning and implication of the claim. This often requires the use of references. Arguments may also include backing in the form of specific incidents, hypothetical scenarios, and personal experiences that illustrate and reinforce the point stated in the claim (Hart, 1998). An example of backing can be found in the literature review about mentoring that was introduced in Box 8.1: the high attrition rate of novice teachers impacts the stability and continuity of schools' culture, and may cause an increased financial burden on school districts.

Counterclaim/Rebuttal

There are very few arguments that do not have competing points of view, a counterapproach, or conflicting evidence. You may also recognize a debate in your field and find yourself a proponent of one position or another.

Building a strong and credible claim requires that you recognize both sides of the argument and respond to a point of view contrary to your own. By doing so, you reinforce the soundness of your argument and show that you formed your position after honest and responsible examination of both sides of the coin. Additionally, comparing and contrasting your position with opposing or alternative argumentations provides an opportunity to clarify or refine your perception (Booth et al., 2008; Hart, 1998).

There are three common ways of counterclaiming and explaining away opposing evidence or alternative point of view:

1. Highlighting the weaknesses and shortcomings in the evidence contained in the counterclaim.

2. Demonstrating the weakness or irrelevancy of the objections presented by those who oppose the approach you advocate.

3. Acknowledging that some of the opposition's arguments have merit and incorporating elements of them into your own claims. At the same time, you may also challenge and dispute other parts of the opposing argument.

Examples of phrasing counterpoints may be:

1. Some researchers (e.g., . . .) disagree with this position on the ground that. . . .

2. There are theoreticians (e.g., . . .) who critique this model and question its merit because. . . .

3. We question the merits of the evidence presented by critics of this approach. For example. . . .

4. While I agree with this researcher on some aspects of her claims, I still see evidence indicating that. . . .

5. Although I disagree with these researchers, they do raise an important issue. . . .

Whichever strategy you follow, it is essential that your presentation of counterpoints is accurate and done with fairness and respect. Never mock or belittle an argument you oppose.

Reasoning Patterns

The discussion above highlighted the elements included in an argument. But, in fact, there are different patterns of argument that vary in the ways they structure the reasons (or evidence) given for reaching conclusions or proposed claims. Following we introduce four patterns with varying levels of complexity: one-on-one reasoning, independent reasoning, dependent reasoning, and chain reasoning (Fisher, 2004; Machi & McEvoy, 2012; Walton, 2013). We briefly describe each pattern, illustrate it with a diagram, and provide an example. While various terminologies are used to describe these reasoning patterns, we follow the terminology offered by Walton (2013).

One-on-One Reasoning

According to this pattern, each evidence-based reason leads to one claimed conclusion. This pattern of reasoning is the most elementary logical structure used in writing a literature review. Visually this pattern can be represented by the following diagram:

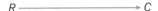

$$R \longrightarrow C$$

where R stands for "reason," C stands for "conclusion," and the arrow stands for "therefore." An example of one-on-one reasoning is presented in Box 8.4.

BOX 8.4. An Example of One-on-One Reasoning

A study by Tessema, Ready, and Astani (2014) investigated the correlation between the average number of hours students worked per week and two dependent variables: student satisfaction (correlation of $r = -.05$) and GPA (correlation of $r = -.13$). The results show that the variable of weekly working hours was negatively correlated with students' satisfaction and GPA.

Source: Tessema, M. T., Ready, K. J., and Astani, M. (2014).

Independent Reasoning

In this pattern, several evidence-based reasons are offered to support a particular claimed conclusion. Each of these reasons independently justifies the claim on its own; however, together they make the conclusion more convincing. This means that R_1, as well as R_2, as well as R_3, and any other reasons, all lead independently to the same conclusion. This pattern is illustrated in the following diagram:

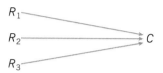

where R_1 stands for Reason 1, R_2 stands for Reason 2, R_3 stands for Reason 3, C stands for "Conclusion," and the arrow stands for "therefore." For an example of independent reasoning, see Box 8.5.

Dependent Reasoning

In this pattern, several evidence-based reasons depend on each other to reach the claimed conclusion. In contrast to the independent pattern, these reasons cannot stand on their own, and a sound conclusion can be drawn only when they are presented jointly. If one of the individual reasons is not plausible or is not supported by credible evidence, the conclusion is not sound. This means that R_1, and R_2, and R_3, and any other additional reasons, are all needed to reach a claimed conclusion. The following diagram illustrates this pattern:

$$R_1 \atop R_2 \atop R_3 \}\ C$$

Coburn and Penuel (2016) may be considered an example of dependent reasoning. This study discusses research–practice partnerships (RPPs), defined as

> **BOX 8.5.** An Example of Independent Reasoning
>
> Many educators and researchers (e.g., Bullough, 2011; Campbell, 2008; Joseph & Efron, 2005; Knowles, Lander, & Hawkin, 2012; Rosenberg, 2015) agree that moral meanings pervade all aspects of teachers' work.

long-term collaborations between practitioners and researchers organized to investigate problems of practice and find solutions for them. In the example highlighted in Box 8.6, the authors provide four interdependent reasons to reach their claimed conclusion.

Chain Reasoning

In this pattern, the conclusion of one claim becomes a premise for the next claim. Thus the argument has several layers, where a claim is supported by an intermediate claim and is used, in turn, to support a further claim. The process continues until the final conclusion is reached. This type of reasoning pattern is often used in

---

BOX 8.6. An Example of Dependent Reasoning

Reasons

R_1: In the field of public health, research found that community leaders who formed partnerships with researchers were more likely to dedicate resources to primary prevention programs. Findings indicated that in comparison to control communities, those that entered these partnerships had a positive impact on young adults, such as lower levels of alcohol and cigarette use and lower number of delinquent behaviors (Brown et al., 2011; Hawkins et al., 2008, 2009).

R_2: In the field of mental health, parents and researchers developed and tested interventions that targeted behavior of elementary-school-age youth. They developed a protocol to study the impact of an intervention to reduce parenting stress and children's oppositional behavior. A random-assignment study found the protocol was successful in achieving these goals (McKay et al., 2011).

R_3: In the field of special needs education, a partnership formed to support care for infant and toddlers at risk for autism spectrum disorders found that its collaborative efforts resulted in enhancement of children's communication and developed parenting skills to support child development (Brookman-Frazee et al., 2012).

R_4: In the field of criminology, a partnership focused on reducing gang violence in Boston resulted in reduced overall levels of youth violence compared to trends in similar cities.

Conclusion

In different fields, interventions developed to solve problems of practice through collaborative partnerships between researchers and practitioners have shown positive outcomes (King et al., 2010; Metzler et al., 2003).

Source: Based on Coburn and Penuel (2016).

theory building. The argument's pattern is $(R_1 + R_2 = C_1)$, then $(C_1 + R_3 = C_2)$, $(C_2 + R_4 = C_3)$, and so on, leading together to the claimed conclusion C. This pattern is represented in the following diagram:

$$R_1 + R_2$$
$$\downarrow$$
$$C_1 + R_3$$
$$\downarrow$$
$$C_2 + R_4$$
$$\downarrow$$
$$C$$

An example of chain reasoning can be found in a study about the value of foster parent care in the context of schooling. In this example (see Box 8.7), there are four layers leading to the claimed conclusion.

Remember, for each pattern of claim you use it is crucial that you construct it logically and that it be supported by research data or by other sources that serve as evidence and substantiate it. The connection between the evidence and the claim should be clear and direct. Additionally, if a warrant that links the evidence to the claim is questionable, you may want to justify it by citing source material.

BOX 8.7. An Example of Chain Reasoning

Argument Layers

1. Kids without a home or abused children suffer from anxiety due to their concerns and worries. This anxiety negatively affects their ability to concentrate. The lack of concentration has detrimental effects on these children's academic achievement (Scherr, 2007).

2. To mitigate these detrimental educational effects, children who are homeless or abused require a stable home that provides a sense of safety and emotional security (Geiger & Schelbe, 2014).

3. Stable homes offer emotional security, stability, and safety. Reliable foster parents provide such homes and thus allow the children to focus on their schoolwork (Frey, 2014; Okpych & Courtney, 2014).

4. The ability to focus on schoolwork allows many students in a stable foster care environment to improve their educational performance (Pecora, Williams, & Kessler, 2005).

Conclusion

Stable foster care often provides significant academic benefits for homeless or abused children.

As you develop the claims that build your literature review's arguments, be sure to avoid fallacious arguments that lead to misleading, mistaken, or untrustworthy conclusions. Based on Hart (1998) and Machi and McEvoy (2012), here are some common mistakes that may hurt the credibility of your argument:

▶ **Unsubstantiated assertions:** Do not substantiate your assertions by using unreliable and unconvincing evidences; rather use trustworthy sources that preferably are available in the public domain.

▶ **Unrelated evidence:** Do not base your conclusions on evidence that is not directly related, relevant, and applicable to the claims you propose.

▶ **Ignoring alternatives:** Do not offer only one interpretation or one explanation as if there are one or more ways to explain or perceive an issue. Present alternative explanations, interpretations, or perceptions.

▶ **Pretended similarities:** Do not claim that two things are similar when there are real differences between them.

▶ **Extremities:** Do not focus only on unusual or extreme ends of a spectrum of alternatives and ignore the more centered position.

▶ **False causality:** Be sure that when you claim a causality, there is an irrefutable connection between the causing action and the resulting effect.

▶ **Implied definition:** Be sure to define the major concepts you refer to in your claim.

▶ **Emotional language:** Avoid using ethically loaded terms or basing your claim on emotional rather than evidence-backed reasons.

▶ **Biased language:** Do not use phrases in a biased way to reinforce your position without providing evidence to support it.

▶ **Personal attacks:** Do not engage in name-calling on a personal level or insult authors with opposing points of view.

GROUP WORK

Choose an argument from your review to share and assess with your group, starting by using the checklist in Table 8.1 (p. 170), and followed by a group discussion.

1. Together with your group, complete the checklist as it relates to the argument or major claim you have written.

2. Group Discussion:
   a. How compelling is your argument and how convincing is your evidence?
   b. Assess how well did you present a position that is different from your own, and how you have responded to it. Did you back each point with evidence?

TABLE 8.1. A Checklist to Assess an Argument Presented in the Literature Review	
	✓
The argument includes:	
■ A claim that justifies the argument	
■ Data that supports the claim	
■ A warrant that links the claim to the evidence	
The claim is:	
■ On point	
■ Precise	
■ Significant	
The evidence is:	
■ Accurate	
■ Precise	
■ Authoritative	
■ Representative	
■ Current	
■ Relevant	
The warrant supports the claim by providing a sound link between the evidence and the claim.	
The claim is stated with qualifiers that define the scope of the conditions under which the claim is true.	
The argument includes:	
■ Definitions or background information	
■ Competing points of view or conflicting evidence	
The reasoning patterns are:	
■ One-on-one	
■ Independent	
■ Dependent	
■ Chain	

Constructing the argument you put forward is a critical ingredient in writing your review of the literature. This is true in the two kinds of arguments mentioned above, the argument of discovery and the argument of advocacy (Machi & McEvoy, 2012).

In the *argument of discovery* you analyze a previous body of work and present what you have discovered while reading the sources about your research subject. The focus is on what is known about your topic. The *argument of advocacy,* which is the closing section of the review, interprets the meaning of that knowledge in the context of future implications.

The role of the argument of advocacy is to summarize the information you have gained through your readings and interpret it in the context of the questions you posed as you introduced your review. Here you also critically assess the current knowledge on your subject and lay the foundations for extending that knowledge. The following section discusses this process and is divided into three parts: (1) summarizing and interpreting what is known, (2) critically evaluating what is known, and (3) extending what is known. As with all facets of the literature review's development, these elements are not permanent or fixed. You are encouraged to structure and present these components according to your review's purpose and your style of writing.

Summarizing and Interpreting What Is Known

In this section you summarize and interpret what you have learned as you develop the argument of discovery. Start by reminding the readers of your original review questions and consider how the knowledge gained through the analysis and synthesis of the literature answered these question. You may do so in a way that captures main themes of your argument, highlights patterns identified, points out major findings, and surveys how the topic has been studied. Tell the readers what meanings and insights you have drawn from the texts and how they correspond to your stated questions. Your interpretations should drive home your research agenda while also being true to the authors you have covered in the review.

The summary should be brief and consist of concise statements. Do not present new information that has not been introduced before or provide conclusions that raise issues not addressed in the body of the review. Some literature review writers like to include bullets or tables to highlight central points they wish to emphasize.

Critically Evaluating What Is Known

As you summarize the overall vigor and robustness of the knowledge gained through your literature review, you also want to assume, once again, a critical stance and evaluate the merits and limitations of the studies done on your topic. You should highlight problems with previous works and identify gaps, contradictions, underrepresentations, or omissions. For example, you may draw attention to the lack or limited amount of research conducted on important aspects of your subject, or point to the fact that certain population groups have been underrepresented or completely ignored. You may also indicate that the methodology used so far does not represent the participants' understanding of the phenomenon or, alternatively, that the scope of the research was limited and therefore the findings may not be generalized to a wider population. Additionally, you may identify the limitations of the theoretical frameworks and conceptualizations of the topic, or highlight contradictions among them.

In quantitative reviews this section offers critical analysis of study design and statistical findings. Issues discussed may include validity and reliability or levels of statistical significance, and major errors and their meanings should be highlighted. The critical discussion may be followed by considerations of how these issues affect the studies' overall findings and conclusions. When it comes to qualitative and hermeneutic–phenomenological reviews, some researchers propose that in addition to the critical assessment of previous studies, the writer should direct the same critical stance toward him- or herself (Douglas, 2014; Wellington et al., 2005). Writers may scrutinize how their theoretical positions and held assumptions impacted their choice of references, the questions asked, and the analysis and interpretations given to current knowledge.

Terms like *need* or *problem* are often used to indicate a critique of the limitations of current research. Some of the most common templates used by literature review writers to introduce critique-indicating elements are:

▶ More research is needed to determine whether. . . .
▶ The problem with current findings is its narrow focus. . . .
▶ There is a clear lack of representation when it comes to. . . .
▶ The problem that surfaced through the review of current research is. . . .
▶ Little is known about how . . . , or the extent to which. . . .

Extending What Is Known

The literature review, asserts Torraco (2005), should serve as a catalyst for extending the current knowledge. An evaluation of existing literature and identification of weaknesses found in the studies reviewed point to aspects that need to be further explored. These aspects may include future research that should be conducted or actions that need to be taken. Depending on whether the literature review is a stand-alone or embedded, these recommendations are directed toward the field in general or provide a rationale for the reviewer's own study.

Stand-Alone Review

In a stand-alone review (see Chapter 1), the discussion of the current knowledge on a particular subject is self-contained and is not intended to be followed by a research study. As the writers reflect on the meaning of the literature, they often recommend actions, such as changes in policy or practice, or they may point out problems and limitations in the reviewed texts. The writers, then, challenge scholars in the field to extend the current knowledge by proposing future lines of inquiry. In Box 8.8, Gunn and Delafield-Butt (2016) conclude their review by recommending change in classroom practice as well as making suggestions for future research.

Embedded Review

In an embedded review the survey of the literature serves as a foundation for a thesis, dissertation, research project, or grant proposal. The writer aims to make a connection between what is known and the research questions that will drive his or her future research study. The critique provides a rationale for the proposed

---

BOX 8.8. An Example of a Discussion in a Stand-Alone Review

In sum, the evidence reviewed in this article indicates substantial benefits in social engagement, learning, and behavior for children with ASD [autism spectrum disorder] when their RIs [restricted interests] are included in classroom practice. Thus we recommend that the RIs of children with ASD be incorporated into the mainstream curriculum where reasonable to do so to facilitate learning and socializing. Intrinsic reward-based methods including integrating the RI into teaching materials or tasks are deemed preferential to extrinsic, consequence-based methods, though either can be successful. . . .

The articles reviewed here represent the sum of our scientific knowledge on RI inclusion in education, but more work needs to be done. Future studies with larger sample sizes testing specific techniques of RI inclusion will afford improved understanding of how children with ASD are motivated by, and can learn through, exploration of their RIs. Knowledge of how RIs affect motivation, self-regulation of interest and learning, and socioemotional well-being will afford insight into the etiology of ASD as well as inform broad educational means for achieving an enjoyable life of learning. A study carried out across various mainstream educational settings, including extracurricular and home environments, could further improve our understanding and the efficacy of this particular inclusive practice.

Source: Gunn and Delafield-Butt (2016).

study by explaining, for example, how the investigation will fill the gap in the existing body of knowledge, resolve current conflicts, or overcome limitations identified in previous research.

The example in Box 8.9 illustrates how Goldhaber, Lavery, and Theobald (2015) claim that their study was designed to make three contributions to existing knowledge by providing missing aspects of current research and building upon it.

An example of the three parts of the final section of the literature review that interpret the meaning of the argument can be found in Box 8.10, taken from a study by Quinn and Cooc (2015). We separated the original text by identifying and labeling in the narrative the Summary, Critique, and Extension of Knowledge sections.

BOX 8.9. An Example of a Rationale for Extending the Existing Knowledge

First, we provide the first comprehensive analysis of the inequitable distribution of both input . . . and output . . . measures of teacher quality across different indicators of student disadvantage . . . using data from a single state.

Second, we decompose these teacher quality gaps into district, school, and classroom effects. To our knowledge, only one prior article (Clotfelter et al., 2005) has done this. . . . Our results provide a broader understanding of the degree to which, at least in one state, inequity is explained by teachers sorting across districts, across schools, within a district, and across classrooms within a school.

Finally, following Sass et al. (2010), we focus on the lower tail of the teacher quality distribution. . . . We build on Sass et al. by considering a full range of student disadvantage indicators, rather than just student poverty level, as well as a full range of teacher quality measures, rather than just value added.

Source: Goldhaber, Lavery, and Theobald (2015).

BOX 8.10. An Example of the Final Section of the Literature Review That Includes Summary, Critical Evaluation, and an Extension of What Is Known

Summary

Developing scientific literacy is an important goal for all students, and disparities in science achievement by gender and race/ethnicity are indicators of educational inequity that can foreshadow other inequities in adulthood. Research has shown that high school students' achievement in STEM predicts whether they will enter and persist in a STEM field in college, and high school STEM achievement helps to explain racial gaps in STEM persistence in college.

(continued)

BOX 8.10. *(continued)*

Critique

This raises questions about how young students' early experiences lay the foundation for these inequalities, yet little is known about how science gaps may develop as a cohort of students progresses through elementary and middle school, or the extent to which early science gaps may be explained by individual factors (such as student SES and prior math and reading achievement) and contextual factors that vary between schools or within school.

Extension of Knowledge

In the study, we address these limitations of the literature by using nationally representative longitudinal data to answer the following questions:

Research Question 1 (RQ1): What are the science test score gaps by gender and race/ethnicity in Grade 3 to Grade 8?

Research Question 2 (RQ2): To what extent do (a) individual factors and (b) schools, teachers, and classrooms explain eighth-grade science test gaps?

Source: Quinn and Cooc (2015).

GROUP WORK

As a group, read the closing sections of each other's literature reviews (argument of discovery), focusing on the following three points: summary and interpretation, critical evaluation, and extending what is known.

1. Consider how well the final section develops these three elements:
   a. Summary and interpretation
      • Answering the original questions
      • Capturing the main theme of the argument
      • Drawing meanings and insights from the proposed argument
   b. Critical evaluation
      • Highlighting problems with previous works
      • Identifying gaps, contractions, underrepresentation, or omissions
   c. Extending what is known
      • Extending the study to a group not investigated before
      • Considering implications for the field
2. Provide feedback and suggestions for improvements, as necessary.
3. Based on group feedback rewrite or revise your final section.

WHAT'S NEXT?

Our discussion in this chapter was divided into two parts: the first one focused on constructing your claims and arguments (argument of discovery); the second one centered on the literature review's final section (argument of advocacy). In the following chapter we describe the process of synthesizing and interpreting different types of sources and offer strategies for doing so.

CHAPTER SUMMARY

1. An argument is the main idea that reflects your standpoint on the topic of your review; it is presented in order to persuade your audience that what you propose is justified.

2. In most literature reviews there are two kinds of basic arguments, referred to as *argument of discovery* and *argument of advocacy*. These two kinds of arguments differ in their goals and in the way they are constructed.

3. Every argument is formed by answering these questions: What is your claim? What evidence justifies your support of the claim? What is the underlying assumption that connects the evidence to your claim?

4. Evidence is data that is used to back up a claim. It should come from empirical (quantitative or qualitative) data, as well as from conceptual, theoretical, or philosophical works written by scholars in your field or in related areas.

5. *Warrant* is a link between the evidence and the claim it is supposed to support. The warrant should ensure that (a) the assumption embedded within the principle is widely regarded as valued among the author's audience, and (b) the logic behind the warrant clearly applies to both the specific claim and the particular evidence that are put forward.

6. Three more components are important for establishing the soundness of a claim: *qualifier, backing,* and *counterclaim*.

7. There are several reasoning patterns that differ from each other in their level of complexity: (a) *one-on-one* reasoning, (b) *independent* reasoning, (c) *dependent* reasoning, and (d) *chain* reasoning.

8. The credibility of your review is compromised by unsubstantiated assertions, unrelated evidence, ignoring alternatives, pretended similarities, extremities, false causality, implied definition, emotional language, biased language, and personal attacks.

9. The *argument of advocacy,* which is the closing section of the review, presents the future implications of the knowledge you gained through the review.

10. The argument of advocacy is often divided into three parts: (a) summarizing and interpreting what is known, (b) critically evaluating what is known, and (c) extending what is known.

Synthesizing and Interpreting the Literature

The focus of the previous chapter was on constructing sound arguments for your literature review that advance or expand what is known and present it from your own unique perspective. The process of systematically laying the claims that build your argument may have seemed a bit mechanistic and prescriptive. However, while building arguments is part of synthesizing and interpreting your sources, the overall process cannot be reduced to mechanical tasks (Britten et al., 2002). A prominent quality of the phase in which you synthesize and interpret your selected literature texts is its creativity and thoughtful search for meaning. At the heart of this process are the original connections you make among your selected sources and the logical linkages you form between them and the literature review questions (Ridley, 2012).

As writers weave together elements from separate texts to form "a new whole" that is "greater than the sum of the constituent parts" (Walsh & Downe, 2005, p. 209), they are using higher-order thinking skills (Dawidowicz, 2010) and a degree of conceptualization (Strike & Posner, 1983). This "new whole" constitutes a holistic story drawn from empirical and theoretical literature on your topic that is synthesized into a cohesive argument (Pope, Mays, & Popay, 2007). Booth et al. (2016) describe this process as using existing blocks to build a new structure.

Synthesizing the sources means bringing together separate elements from the individual studies or pieces of evidence and weaving them logically together to produce a coherent whole in the form of an argument, a theory, or a conclusion (Pope et al., 2007). There are two main forms of synthesis: aggregative and interpretative. *Aggregative synthesis* focuses on collecting and summarizing multiple studies in order to accumulate knowledge and look for generalizable conclusions. This form of synthesis, although used at times for traditional–narrative review, is mostly used for the synthesis of quantitative studies and systematic reviews (Dixon-Woods et al., 2006b). *Interpretative synthesis* brings existing studies together in a creative manner in order to develop new concepts, arguments, explanations, or theories. The writer adopting this approach uses inventive techniques to maximize the explanatory value of the data (Dixon-Woods et al., 2006b). This approach has mostly been associated with synthesis of qualitative and hermeneutic–phenomenological studies (Noblit & Hare, 1988).

In this chapter, we describe the process of synthesizing and interpreting the literature. We start by highlighting the strategies that are used in traditional–narrative synthesis. These strategies are often used by reviewers of other types of research as well. We then highlight those strategies that are unique to the synthesis of quantitative, qualitative, mixed-methods, and hermeneutic–phenomenological studies.

SYNTHESIS OF TRADITIONAL–NARRATIVE LITERATURE

Synthesizing the literature about your topic around a cohesive line of argumentation requires moving the analysis of individual sources to a "higher level of abstraction, subsuming the particulars into the general" (Whittemore & Knafl, 2005, p. 551). To achieve this higher level of abstraction, you need to make connections among the individual sources you consult while researching your topic and look for patterns and trends.

There are several strategies that may enhance your ability to systematically recognize emerging patterns and trends within the sea of information: grouping the sources, comparing and contrasting the sources, exploring conflicting or contradicting findings, and adopting critical dispositions. As stated above, while we list the strategies under traditional–narrative synthesis, you may find them applicable in other types of syntheses.

GROUPING THE SOURCES

You may refer back to your sources, revisit your article note-taking index cards (ANTICs) and thematic concentric circles (see Chapter 5), and refer to the themes and subthemes that you identified as you developed the architectural structures of your sources (matrix, tables, maps, and outline; see Chapter 7). The organizational structure you have developed will help you to discern the relationships within and among the variables, themes, constructs, and patterns you have identified and determine how they intersect (Booth et al., 2016). The connections you make between the multiple ideas, concepts, methodologies, and pieces of evidence need to be "coherent and explicit" (Hart, 1998, p. 111). This entails being continuously aware of the whole while you are examining the specific components—and all the while considering how both are related to the questions that guide your literature review.

For example, let's go back to the literature review written by Eric, the middle school principal whose research is focused on charter schools. He looks back at the ANTICs, the thematic concentric circles, and the synthesis matrix he created and groups studies according to themes such as differences in middle school students' standardized test scores, school curriculum, school organizational structure, and parent involvement, as well as the particular research methodologies used in the included studies.

Comparing and Contrasting Sources

Once you group the studies around variables, concepts, or themes, the next step is to determine how the studies are connected, related, or differ from each other. One useful way to examine the relationships among the concepts, ideas, and variables within the themes is through engaging in a process of comparing and contrasting groups of data. This exercise enables you to identify similarities and differences among diverse studies, such as different theories, policies, alternative methodologies, research designs, and various findings and conclusions. Moreover, it helps you discern whether the findings or positions support, reinforce, or contrast with each other. This process also allows you to recognize the complexities and nuances of the topic, and to realize that even though a group of studies may seem to be homogenous, there could be areas of variation (Booth et al., 2016).

A Venn diagrams is one of the best methods to graphically compare and contrast the ideas, theories, methodologies, and research findings discussed in your source materials (Hart, 1998; Machi & McEvoy, 2012). To create a Venn diagram, simply draw overlapping circles. Each circle represents a theoretical, methodological, or empirical body of work. In the central overlapping area, list the common elements; in the areas outside of the intersection note those aspects that differentiate the two data sets.

To illustrate the use of a Venn diagram, let's go back to the literature review written by Eric on charter schools. A central theme of his literature review distinguishes charter public schools (CPS) from traditional public schools (TPS). Eric realized that a Venn diagram would be helpful in comparing the two types of schools and decided to incorporate it into his writing of the literature review. Figure 9.1 (p. 180) depicts the diagram he constructed to compare the two types of schools.

When creating a Venn diagram, you need to ensure that the claims of commonalities and differences are valid and verifiable. For example, you cannot claim that charter schools always perform better than traditional public schools if you do

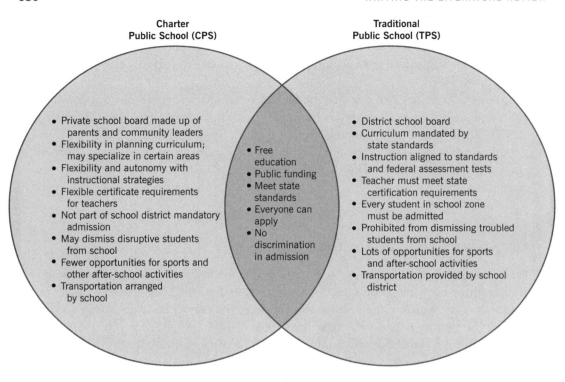

FIGURE 9.1. A Venn diagram comparing charter and traditional public schools.

not have evidence to support such a statement. Additionally, an appropriate set of criteria or points of comparison must be meaningful and comparable. Hart (1998) points out that even though it is an essential aspect for the process of comparison, rarely can all elements on one side be matched with comparable elements on the other side.

In Boxes 9.1, 9.2, and 9.3 (p. 181), we offer examples of three sets of criteria for comparing and contrasting sources. Box 9.1 centers on contrasting two or three theories. Boxes 9.2 and 9.3, which are based on Dawidowicz's (2010) suggestions, offer two sets of criteria for comparing and contrasting quantitative and qualitative studies of a phenomena. Box 9.2 presents criteria for quantitative studies and Box 9.3 presents criteria for qualitative or hermeneutical studies.

Exploring Conflicting or Contradictory Findings

As you juxtapose different sources, your natural tendency might be to find comprehensive or cohesive explanations, patterns, or conclusions. Like many review writers, Eric's first tendency was to identify similarities and repeating relationships

BOX 9.1. Comparing and Contrasting Theories

1. What is the major goal of each theory?
2. What is the central claim of each theory?
3. Who are the theoreticians or researchers most associated with the theory?
4. How does the theory apply to the social/economic/policy aspects of your field?
5. What are the practical implications of the theory?
6. What are the main points of criticism of this theory?

BOX 9.2. Criteria for Comparing and Contrasting Quantitative Studies

Are there similarities or differences in:

1. Theoretical framework?
2. Research assumptions?
3. Research design?
4. Research sample?
5. Research results?
6. Research conclusions?
7. Research limitations?

BOX 9.3. Criteria for Comparing and Contrasting Qualitative or Hermeneutical Studies

Are there similarities of differences in:

1. Theoretical framework?
2. Historical background?
3. Setting's socioeconomic conditions?
4. Culture of the setting?
5. Individuals (or organizations) involved?
6. Participants' perceived values?
7. Research findings?

in data before he recognized inconsistencies, discordance, and dissonance. It may be tempting for review writers to include only information that confirms their position, explain away conflicting data, or pretend that uncomfortable evidence does not exist. They do so in order to illustrate homogeneity and consistency in their line of argument even when they are presented with a more complex and nuanced reality. However, looking back at the literature, Eric found contradictory findings regarding the performance of public schools when compared with charter schools that he has an obligation to include.

Literature review experts (Booth et al., 2016; Walsh & Downe, 2005; Whittemore & Knafl, 2005) warn reviewers against establishing premature patterns or arguments without challenging them. They contend that such a practice presents a threat to the integrity of the literature review and to the credibility of its claims. The synthesis process, they emphasize, should be transparent; and deviant data, contradicting findings, or rival explanations should be revealed. As was declared by Whittemore and Knafl (2005, p. 551), "Analytical honesty is a priority."

Additionally, as you continue with your reading, revisit and reexamine your initial assertions. You may want to validate them or, alternatively, revise them to ensure that they accurately reflect the information gained from the new texts as well (Booth et al., 2016; Miles, Huberman, & Saldaña, 2013).

When it comes to quantitative data, conflicting results may become a considerable challenge in the synthesis process, especially when the evidence is drawn from equally high-quality studies (Whittemore & Knafl, 2005). To analyze conflicting data, Cooper (1998) suggests using a "vote counting" strategy for finding out the frequency of significant positive findings in comparison to the frequency of significant negative ones. If conflicting evidence persists, the researcher may suggest the need for further research to investigate the issue with a design specifically constructed to resolve this particular conflict.

Researchers might also consider the need to explore study components, such as sample characteristics and research designs, that may have influenced and contributed to variability in findings. Such conflicting evidence often provides an impetus for further investigations (Whittemore & Knafl, 2005). Booth et al. (2016) raise the possibility of an outlier study whose findings in many respects differ markedly from those reported by other researchers who conducted studies on the same topic. In such a case, Booth et al. recommend that the writer decide whether this particular study should be included in the literature review's general analysis or be analyzed separately.

By comparison, in qualitative or hermeneutic–phenomenological studies, deviant data is often welcomed. In fact, absence of differences and contradictions among the sources may cause some suspicion as to the rigor of the analysis and synthesis process, as studies in this approach seldom result in a complete congruence of meanings (Walsh & Downe, 2005). It is crucial, according to Walsh and Downe, not to overlook or ignore differences, but rather view them as an opportunity to gain a more nuanced understanding of a phenomenon and to discover new meanings that were not considered before.

Adopting a Critical Stance

An essential requirement for conducting a quality synthesis of the literature on your topic is carrying it out with a critical stance. The literature review's aim is to provide a critique rather than a mere summary of the readings you have chosen. As Douglas (2014, p. 140) points out, just reporting these sources is "knowledge telling," whereas in your literature review you want to attain "knowledge transforming" and new insight through a critique of the reviewed texts.

The critique of sources is dynamic and recursive; it occurs at different points of the literature review process. As you remember, we previously discussed in-depth ways to evaluate the quality of individual research articles (see Chapter 6). At the synthesis phase, as you bring together the materials from different sources to create an integrated whole, you move from a critical appraisal of individual studies to critiquing the body of literature as a whole. Ridley (2012, p. 141) uses the term "critical reading" to define the stage of evaluating individual texts and distinguishes it from the "critical writing" that takes place during the phase of literature synthesis.

At the critical writing phase, your individual evaluations are woven together and synthesized around the major themes and central arguments that you put forward. In this phase, you shed light on the strengths and shortcomings of the studies. For example, Jennifer, a doctoral student in psychology, conducted a mixed-methods study about social skills among teenagers. In her literature review, one of the themes in her discussion was the effect of the Internet on the development of interpersonal relationships. In reviewing the studies conducted on this theme, she presented findings by different authors who explored young people's perspectives using interviews and surveys to find out how Internet use enhances or weakens their ability to authentically communicate with each other. As part of her review, Jennifer highlighted the strengths and limitations of the methodologies used by the researchers and their effects on the validity and trustworthiness of the studies' findings.

It is especially advisable to critique the different sources together when you identify patterns of strengths and weaknesses that are common across these studies. You may offer more in-depth criticism of selected sources that are especially important to your own research focus or those studies that are often referred to in your narrative.

Being critical requires you to read the texts closely, scrutinize them carefully, critique evidence, appraise methodologies, and explore the processes by which the researchers reach their conclusions. In your critique you consider the soundness of studies applicable to your topic and assess the validity of the arguments put forward by the researchers. You may point out the shortcomings of the arguments by highlighting fallacies, inadequacies, limitations of evidence, or lack of plausibility (Hart, 1998). It is also advisable to focus the critique on the major critical points rather than on minor or insignificant details. Additionally, when wtriting qualitative and hermeneutic–phenomenological reviews, the criticism may be directed at "problematizing" the current discourse in the field and challenging the nature of the assumptions that underlie it (Boell & Cecez-Kecmanovic, 2014; Dixon-Woods et al., 2006b).

You should assume a critical stance and even question the works of leading academics. Your evaluation should be informed, deliberate, respectful, and fair; the critique should not misrepresent or misinterpret the source texts but rather be based on what is actually reported in them (Wellington et al., 2005). It is not enough to simply offer a list of deficiencies or just state that a study's findings or theoretical propositions are inadequate or weak. Instead, your criticism should provide a clear explanation of what is wrong with the theory or study's conclusions and present convincing reasons for your assessment.

Being critical requires an openness to the different or even contrasting modes of understanding (Wellington et al., 2005); it obliges you to be deliberate, reflexive, and confident, while at the same time humble and respectful. Most importantly, it necessitates that your judgment be fair and balanced.

Elbow (1973) reinforces this position by arguing that when writing a critique of your sources you need to balance the "believing" and "doubting" phases. In the *believing* phase, you intentionally open yourself to the writers' points of view and try to understand their claims and ideas from their perspectives. On the other hand, the *doubting* phase entails adopting a skeptical and questioning stance and approaching the texts critically. Together, the two approaches allow you to review the literature rigorously and recognize complexities and multiple layers within your topic.

To summarize, the common strategies used in synthesizing traditional–narrative studies are grouping the sources, comparing and contrasting the sources, exploring conflicting or contradictory findings, and adopting a critical stance. Figure 9.2 illustrates these common strategies.

We described the strategies that are used in traditional–narrative synthesis and stated that they may be applicable to other types of reviews. However, there are also differences in how the synthesis process is perceived in quantitative, qualitative, mixed-methods, and hermeneutic–phenomenological studies. Therefore, each of these types of studies may require distinctive methods of analysis and synthesis. Following is a brief discussion that highlights the features that distinguish each of these approaches.

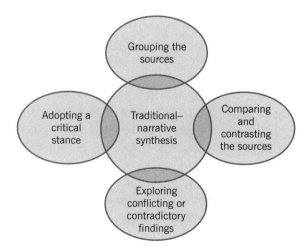

FIGURE 9.2. Common strategies that characterize the traditional–narrative literature synthesis.

|||||||||||||||||||||||||||||||||||||||||||||||||||||||||||||||||||||||||||**SYNTHESIS OF QUANTITATIVE LITERATURE**

Synthesizing quantitative sources in relation to the study's research questions allows literature review writers to discover and explain relationships among variables (Booth et al., 2016) and assess the internal and external validity of each study. (See Chapter 6 for a discussion of internal and external validity.) When selecting quantitative sources for inclusion in your analysis, you should determine the quality of each source. The selection criteria should be applied vigorously and consistently to ensure that studies selected meet the inclusion criteria and that you do not overlook or ignore relevant studies. Criteria should also be clear and objective so that someone else who is using them would choose the same studies (McDonald, 2014). (See Chapter 5 for our discussion of inclusion and exclusion criteria.)

There are two popular approaches you can use to synthesize the quantitative data in studies you found on your topic: meta-analysis and quantitative narrative (Schick-Makaroff, MacDonald, Plummer, Burgess, & Neander, 2016). *Meta-analysis* refers to the use of statistical procedures to combine, analyze, and synthesize numerical data from individual studies that are focused on the same topic or research question. Meta-analysis combines statistical findings from multiple studies, thereby yielding results that individual studies cannot offer (Lau, Ioannidis, & Schmid, 1997). By comparison, *quantitative narrative synthesis* is a systematic review that is more intuitive, and refers to a summary and synthesis of results from multiple studies that include quantitative data by using words and text. Both of these approaches provide a systematic process for drawing conclusions that are orderly and can be subjected to audit (Petticrew & Roberts, 2006; Schick-Makaroff et al., 2016). We discuss both approaches to synthesizing quantitative literature in the sections that follow.

Meta-Analysis

The term *meta-analysis* was first used by Glass in 1976 (p. 3). Although studies that statistically combine multiple studies were undertaken beginning in the early 1900s, meta-analysis was rarely used in the social sciences before the 1970s (Cooper et al., 2009). This approach allows researchers to study the effect of an intervention, treatment, or program across multiple studies and to determine the size of the effect using findings from multiple primary research studies. When researchers combine data from multiple studies, the sample size is larger than that of a single study (Jesson et al., 2011). Unlike a traditional literature review that depends on the reviewer's own interpretation of the research, meta-analysis uses more objective and rigorous statistical methods to combine, analyze, and synthesize multiple sources of data on the topic of interest. Meta-analysis is also used to chart a new direction for future research (Schmidt & Hunter, 2015).

To illustrate the use of meta-analysis in research, we can look at the study conducted by Melinda, a doctoral student in psychology, whose research on childhood depression was introduced earlier (see Chapter 3). As part of her literature review, she conducted a meta-analysis to analyze outcomes of intervention programs that were undertaken to alleviate childhood depression symptoms. She uses the findings to plan her own research on this topic.

Many review writers may find it difficult to carry out a meta-analysis due to the fact that it requires a higher level of knowledge of statistics. Nevertheless, we concur with Pan (2013), who argues that all review writers—those writing quantitative or qualitative reviews—should understand the basics of meta-analysis in order to understand and interpret studies using this method if they find them in the literature they are reviewing.

Effect Size

Effect size is an index that is used to show a *difference* between two means, such as those obtained in a study comparing treatment and control groups (R. Ravid, 2015). It can also be used to express the magnitude of an *association* between two variables using a correlation coefficient. This can be done by converting the correlation coefficient—the index of the strength of the association—into an effect size (R. Ravid, 2015). Converting study data into an effect size can be done first for each study included in the analysis; the studies are then combined for the meta-analysis procedure. Comparing the results of the meta-analysis by using a diagram is also an effective way to examine the results from multiple studies (Jesson et al., 2011).

Box 9.4 shows how the effect size was calculated in a study conducted to assess the relationships among the constructs of acculturation, enculturation, and acculturation strategies (Yoon et al., 2013).

BOX 9.4. An Example of the Calculation of Effect Size (ES)

The correlation coefficient, r, was the ES measure of choice for most analyses. A few ESs (4.5%), including other statistics (e.g., means and standard deviations, t tests), were converted to r. The only analyses that used means and standard deviations without conversions to r were conducted to estimate mean differences in mental health between integration and other acculturation strategies (i.e., assimilation, separation, and marginalization).

Source: Yoon et al. (2013).

Publication Bias

Publication bias can occur when the sample of studies chosen to be included in the analysis is biased and thus presents a threat to the validity of the results (Rothstein, Sutton, & Borenstein, 2005). (See Chapter 5 for a discussion of publication bias.) Although it is of concern in all types of research reviews, it is more of a concern in meta-analysis because it can skew the results of the analysis. Publication bias can be addressed by researchers conducting meta-analyses through the use of statistical procedures to correct for potential publication bias (Card, 2015).

Meta-analysis is usually undertaken with a team of at least two researchers to confirm the selection of studies to be included. Using agreed-upon inclusion and exclusion criteria, these researchers review studies and decide whether to include them in the analysis. The process of choosing studies using more than one researcher helps establish interrater reliability. Additionally, the research team should ensure that the data from the different studies that are combined for the meta-analysis are free of computational errors, there are no missing cases, and similar groups (on variables such as age and treatments) are combined in the analysis. Uman (2011) recommends that these researchers keep a log of all the studies they reviewed, clearly indicating reasons for excluding certain studies or including others in the meta-analysis.

Outliers

Outliers can also present a problem in meta-analysis. Outliers are studies that report a data set that is clearly very different from the rest of the data on that topic. Outliers can be especially problematic when the number of studies for the meta-analysis is small, as they can greatly influence the outcome of the analysis. Researchers should explore the possible reasons for the presence of outliers, such as issues related to the study design or mistakes in data computations. Researchers have developed a variety of statistical methods designed to deal with the potential problem of outliers (e.g., Viechtbauer & Cheung, 2010); however, these are beyond the scope of this discussion.

TO DO: *How to Synthesize Data Using Meta-Analysis*

Table 9.1 (p. 188) lists the major steps involved in synthesizing data using meta-analysis. These steps follow a comprehensive search of the literature and selection of studies for inclusion using strict agreed-upon criteria.

TABLE 9.1. Steps for Synthesizing Data Using Meta-Analysis
Step
1. Extract the data from the chosen studies.
2. Choose an appropriate common outcome measure (effect size) to represent the data from each of the studies.
3. Apply a statistical method to combine all the included studies and compute the appropriate effect size across the studies.
4. Display the meta-analysis results using a graphic presentation that displays data from individual studies, as well as the pooled estimate.
5. Interpret the findings.

Figure 9.3 (p. 189) illustrates the major steps in searching, analyzing, and synthesizing data using meta-analysis.

The computation of meta-analysis is beyond the scope of this book and requires an advanced knowledge of statistics. Those interested can utilize software programs and consult books that focus on this topic.

Quantitative Narrative Synthesis

Although a quantitative narrative synthesis may lack the power of meta-analysis, it can be the method of choice for reviewers who cannot undertake a meta-analysis. It can also be used to synthesize quantitative studies that cannot be included in a meta-analysis because they do not meet the eligibility criteria. For each study covered, the narrative synthesis includes a discussion of the type of study, a description of the participants, a description of the intervention or study's outcomes, and a critical analysis of the quality of the study. The use of tables can provide an effective way to summarize this information about each study (Ridley, 2012). (You may also use the ANTICs and summary tables discussed in Chapters 5 and 7.)

As a reviewer, you should highlight the heterogeneity of the studies (differences across the studies), identify observed patterns and trends, and comment on the quality of the studies. A short summary of the results of your review should also be provided (Dykiert, 2014; Petticrew & Roberts, 2006).

The process of "vote counting" (mentioned earlier in this chapter) also can be incorporated as a preliminary step in the narrative synthesis process (Ridley, 2012). In addition to using it where there are conflicting results, it can also be applied where there is a limited amount of information reported. Basically, vote counting is done by sorting studies into three categories: (1) studies that report significant positive results (confirming the predicted hypothesis); (2) studies that report

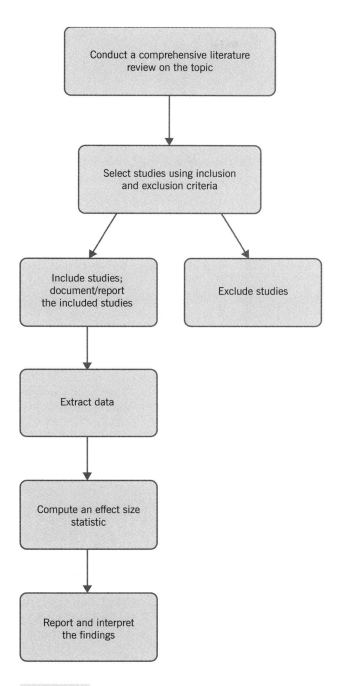

FIGURE 9.3. The major steps in a meta-analysis process.

significant results that are opposite to what was predicted; and (3) studies that report insignificant results (Koricheva & Gurevitch, 2013). However, Koricheva and Gurevitch caution against the use of vote counting, which has several methodological weaknesses, including giving equal weight to studies with small samples and studies with large samples, and the inability to represent the magnitude of the effect reported.

TO DO: How to Create a Narrative Synthesis of Quantitative Data

In the synthesis process, the goal is to organize the sources and group studies with common characteristics in order to compare and contrast them. Petticrew and Roberts (2006) suggest the three steps listed in Table 9.2.

TABLE 9.2. Steps for Creating a Narrative Synthesis of Quantitative Data	
Step	✓
1. Organize the studies using logical categories, such as type of intervention, type of population, or study design. This can be done using tables or in a narrative form organized by categories determined by the reviewer. (See our discussion of ANTICs in Chapter 5.)	
2. Analyze the findings reported *within* each study, adding comments about the study's quality, when appropriate. (See Quantitative Summary table in Chapter 7.)	
3. Synthesize the findings across all the studies that are included in the narrative.	

SYNTHESIS OF QUALITATIVE LITERATURE

There are diverse approaches to the synthesis of qualitative studies, among them meta-ethnography, meta-synthesis, critical interpretive synthesis, and thematic analysis (Barnett-Page & Thomas, 2009; Dixon-Woods et al., 2006a; Lee, Hart, Watson, & Rapley, 2015). All these approaches have their roots in the interpretive–qualitative tradition. They all aim to increase the understanding of a phenomenon by transforming findings of individual qualitative studies into an overarching conceptualization or even conceptualizing a new theory (Polit & Beck, 2013).

Barnett-Page and Thomas (2009) assert that most of these interpretive approaches show similarities in their synthesis approach. Meta-ethnography is considered the most developed and most practiced synthesis approach by many qualitative researchers (Atkins et al., 2008; Britten et al., 2002; Campbell et al., 2003, 2011; Onwuegbuzie & Frels, 2016). Therefore, we are focusing on this approach in our discussion of interpretive synthesis of qualitative studies.

Meta-Ethnography

Meta-ethnography is an inductive and interpretative method of synthesizing research findings. This process involves comparing concepts across individual studies in a belief that it is possible to bring together and synthesize themes and concepts that were identified in different qualitative studies. Essentially, the goal of this process is to create a new and deeper understanding by discovering explicit connections between individual studies that were not visible before (Campbell et al., 2003; Suri, 2011). This process is referred to by Noblit and Hare (1998, p. 28) as "making a whole into something more than the parts alone imply."

Meta-ethnography was originally pioneered by Noblit and Hare (1988) as a process of synthesizing findings of qualitative studies in the field of education. For these researchers, meta-ethnography begins with the premise that all interpretive exploration is "essentially translation" (p. 7). Translation, from this perspective, bridges different qualitative studies by constantly comparing metaphors, concepts, and constructs that represent major themes in the documents. This iterative process allows a progressive discovery of overarching metaphors, concepts, and constructs to emerge (Forte, 2010).

Noblit and Hare provided a description of the analysis-synthesis process that still serves as a framework for current reviewers of qualitative research who follow the meta-ethnography approach today. They proposed three paths in which the translation synthesis across studies may occur: *reciprocal, refutational,* and *line of arguments*. These three types of translation are not distinct from each other but rather are intermingling parts of an iterative, interpretative process (Toye et al., 2014).

Reciprocal synthesis involves the establishment of common concepts and terminology that are used in different studies when describing the same phenomenon. These common overarching concepts are captured through a systematic comparison of papers; the comparison leads to a determination of when metaphors, terms, concepts, or themes from one study match those of another. These terms or metaphors that express comparable concepts or themes may be identical (i.e., direct translation) or different.

Refutational synthesis involves exploring and explaining differences in conflicting interpretations or opposing arguments. The refutational (negative) comparison designed to discern conflicts in data is crucial for comprehensive and nuanced understanding of the topic.

Line of argument synthesis involves analyzing and synthesizing the studies in ways that "put together the similarities and differences between studies into an interpretative logical order" (Noblit & Hare, 1988, p. 64). This process successively builds an overarching interpretation that creates a holistic picture of the whole from the study of its parts (Toye et al., 2014).

While the meta-ethnography synthesis process is done systematically, it is also very intuitive and creative. These intuitive and creative characteristics resist an explicit description of how qualitative analysis and synthesis are done and make full transparency of the process impossible (Campbell et al., 2011).

Still, based on our and other researchers' experiences, we offer commonly used steps practiced in the synthesis process. Since movement from step to step is iterative rather than linear, we recommend experimenting with these suggestions and adapting them to your own specific circumstances, needs, and style.

TO DO: *How to Create a Meta-Ethnography Synthesis*

Table 9.3 is based on the seven steps of synthesis (Noblit & Hare, 1988) as interpreted by several leading researchers in the field (e.g., Atkins et al., 2008; Booth et al., 2016; Britten et al., 2002; Campbell et al., 2011; Doyle, 2003; Forte, 2010; Lee et al., 2015; Walsh & Downe, 2005).

TABLE 9.3. Steps for Creating a Meta-Ethnography Synthesis
Step
1. Identify major metaphors, constructs, and concepts in each study and chart them in a matrix, typically using the terminology of the original paper.
2. Expand the matrix and record the contextual information from each paper and its author's interpretations of the findings.
3. Note areas of convergence through constant comparison and juxtaposition across studies.
4. Refine, progressively, the major metaphors, constructs, or concepts and choose those that most adequately represent the entire data.
5. Review each paper again for the presence or absence of your chosen central concepts and metaphors and identify competing or contradicting ones.
6. Examine central concepts and interpretations and look for building blocks (patterns and themes) that best explain the data from your perspective.
7. Use the patterns and themes as building blocks to construct an integrated account of the phenomenon and develop a cohesive, synthesized argument.

Figure 9.4 (p. 193) illustrates the major steps in searching, analyzing, and synthesizing data using a meta-ethnography process.

The meta-ethnographic process is considered a laborious and intensive endeavor. Campbell et al. (2011) suggest that this method is suited for a synthesis of a smaller number of studies, limited to no more than 40. Otherwise, they propose, the review writers will not be able to gain a "sufficient familiarity" (p. 60) or maintain the high level of rigor that the synthesis work requires.

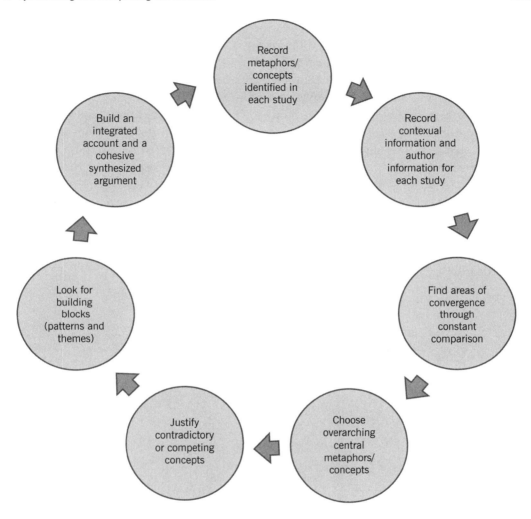

FIGURE 9.4. Meta-ethnography synthesis steps.

Additionally, it is important to note that while the translational activity described above is an interpretative process, the reviewer's interpretation is not based on primary data collected by the researchers, such as interviews and observations. Rather, it is grounded in the interpretations offered by the researchers of the studies and thus is an "interpretation of interpretations" (Forte, 2010, p. 154). This process is similar to Schutz's (1967) conceptualization of first- and second-order constructs. The *first-order construct* refers to the study's data, while the *second-order construct* represents the study researcher's interpretation of that data. In meta-ethnographic literature review, the writers develop an additional level of interpretation, a *third-order construct*. At this level, the review writers present their own independent interpretations of the researchers' interpretations of their studies' findings (Britten, 2002; Lee et al., 2015; Toye et al., 2014).

An example of a third-order construct can be seen in a study conducted by Antony, a sociology doctoral student. He explored issues related to the cultural integration of immigrants who have lived in the United States for the past 10 to 15 years. In his meta-ethnographic review, Antony included data from ethnographic studies that were mostly based on long-term observations and in-depth interviews (first-order construct). During the synthesis process, Antony looked for common themes in the interpretation of the findings as presented by the researchers of the studies he reviewed (second-order construct). Consequently, he discovered connections and relationships between the researchers' findings and was able to gain a holistic understanding of the challenges, frustrations, and successes involved in the process of becoming culturally integrated into the new society (third-order construct).

Figure 9.5 illustrates the process of interpreting researchers' interpretations in third-order constructs.

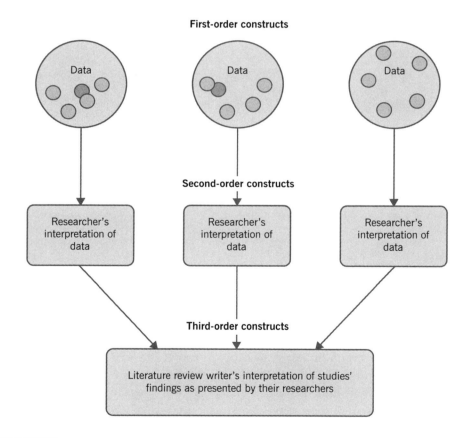

FIGURE 9.5. An illustration of the third-order construct process: interpretation of interpretations.

The issue of third-order constructs points to the tension faced by meta-ethnographic reviewers when trying to find a balance between retaining the original texts and synthesizing the previous sources into an integrative argument (Doyle, 2003). On one hand, there is a desire to maintain the cultural and social contexts of the original texts and represent their perspectives on the phenomenon. At the same time, the reviewer aims toward gaining a holistic understanding and reaching a higher level of theoretical perspective through a synthesis of the previous studies (Britten et al., 2002; Doyle, 2003; Walsh & Downe, 2005).

SYNTHESIS OF MIXED-STUDIES LITERATURE

After discussing methods of synthesizing qualitative and quantitative studies, let's turn to a method of synthesis that brings together quantitative, qualitative, and mixed-methods sources within a single literature review. This method promotes the inclusion of different types of research sources by integrating their findings in order to address the same, overlapping, or complementary questions (Harden & Thomas, 2010).

The term *mixed-methods review* is usually associated with this literature synthesis approach (Hannes, 2015; Harden & Thomas, 2005); however, we agree with Pluye and Hong's (2014) suggestion that this term may lead to a false assumption that this type of synthesis includes only mixed-methods studies. In reality, it includes studies with diverse designs: quantitative, qualitative, and mixed-methods. Therefore, the term *synthesis of mixed studies review* is more appropriate, and we are using it in our discussion here.

There are researchers (e.g., Brannen, 2005; Flick, 2009; Hammersley, 2000; Johnson & Onwuegbuzie, 2004) who maintain that the differences between the theories and methods of quantitative and qualitative approaches are very significant; therefore, they reject the possibility of synthesizing the two approaches in a single literature review. They also claim that since it is easier to synthesize quantitative data, the qualitative data is often relegated to a secondary or supportive role in a mixed-studies approach. Still, since the number of researchers who use both quantitative and qualitative methods in their research has increased greatly in the last decades, there is a growing awareness of the value of mixing the types of studies included in a literature review (Hammersley, 2000; Johnson & Onwuegbuzie, 2004; Saini & Shlonsky, 2012).

According to proponents of mixed-studies synthesis, the combination of quantitative, qualitative, and mixed-methods studies in the review allows the writer to take advantage of the "power of stories with the power of numbers" (Pluye & Hong, 2014, p. 29). For example, qualitative synthesis of participants' subjective perspectives on a program, policy, or intervention may complement the quantitative synthesis of statistical outcomes.

Several methods are often suggested for synthesizing qualitative, quantitative, and mixed-methods studies. According to Heyvaert, Maes, and Onghena (2013), mixed-methods studies reviewers should consider three elements as they synthesize studies:

1. Where is the emphasis placed? Are either qualitative or quantitative methods given a priority or are the two equal?

2. What type of integration is used? Are the data synthesized concurrently or sequentially?

3. What is the degree of integration? Is there a full or parallel integration of the findings?

To these three elements, Pluye and Hong (2014) add a fourth question regarding the mode of analysis and synthesis.

4. Is the mode of analysis and synthesis designed for theory building (exploratory) or theory testing (explanatory)?

The four most common types of mixed-studies synthesis designs that we outline here are based on these four elements. These main designs are segregated synthesis, sequential exploratory synthesis, sequential explanatory synthesis, and convergent synthesis. We briefly describe each of these synthesis designs and offer an example that illustrates the distinct elements of each. Our descriptions, as well as the visual displays of the different design patterns, are based on Pluye and Hong (2014).

Segregated Synthesis

The most basic form of mixed-studies synthesis design is done in two phases. In the first phase, the syntheses of quantitative and qualitative studies are conducted separately. This is followed by a second phase where those syntheses are linked together in the conclusion stage to form a "third synthesis" (Harden & Thomas, 2005). This approach draws from an understanding that qualitative and quantitative studies differ from each other and, therefore, to keep the integrity of the synthesis, the reviewer should use the synthesis methods that are unique to each of these approaches. The separate syntheses then come together and triangulate each other's findings to reach a common conclusion (Sandelowski, Voils, & Barroso, 2006). Figure 9.6 (p. 197) illustrates the process of segregated synthesis.

An example of segregated synthesis was carried out by Alex for the literature review chapter in his doctoral dissertation in sociology. He performed his synthesis using quantitative and qualitative studies to evaluate a new policy used for regulating for-profit colleges. For the quantitative synthesis, Alex conducted a statistical

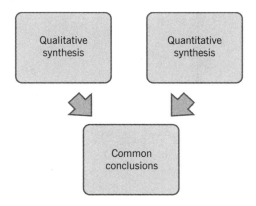

FIGURE 9.6. The process of segregated synthesis.

meta-analysis of studies that explored the economic outcomes of the policy on students enrolled in for-profit colleges. For the qualitative set of studies, he employed strategies of meta-ethnography synthesis in order to examine the perceptions of the students involved regarding the impact of the new policy on their educational experience. The separate syntheses of the quantitative and qualitative studies provided Alex with two sets of findings that he then compared and contrasted in a third synthesis to reach the study's conclusion.

Sequential Exploratory Synthesis

In this two-phase synthesis design, the qualitative synthesis is followed by and contributes to the second phase of the quantitative synthesis. In the first phase, the researcher synthesizes qualitative data, whereas in the second phase (quantitative), these qualitative findings are summarized and tabulated quantitatively in order to test or generalize the findings of the qualitative synthesis (Pluye & Hong, 2014). The purpose of sequential exploratory synthesis is usually to generate a new hypothesis, develop an emerging theory, or identify knowledge gaps. Figure 9.7 (p. 198) illustrates the process of sequential exploratory synthesis.

An example of a sequential exploratory synthesis design is a literature review written by Rosalina, a graduate student in communication, on the impact of computer games on the social communication of young adults. In the first phase of the synthesis process, Rosalina used analysis and synthesis of primary qualitative studies to identify key categories. In the second phase, these categories were measured and appraised to test the qualitative findings and to generalize the results.

Sequential Explanatory Synthesis

In this two-phase synthesis design, the quantitative synthesis is followed by and informs the qualitative synthesis. In phase 1 (quantitative), the numerical

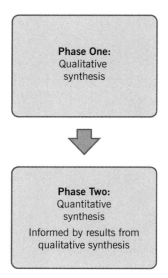

FIGURE 9.7. The process of sequential exploratory synthesis design.

findings from quantitative and mixed-methods studies are analyzed. In phase 2 the quantitative findings from phase 1 are used to interpret the qualitative findings from qualitative and mixed-methods studies. The purpose of sequential explanatory synthesis is to reveal new explanations and highlight gaps in current knowledge. Figure 9.8 (p. 199) illustrates the process of sequential explanatory synthesis.

An example of a sequential explanatory synthesis design is a literature review written by Jackie, a curriculum development specialist for a state board of education. The topic of her research was the effectiveness of the use of multiple-choice tests in assessing high school students' knowledge in social studies. In phase 1 (quantitative), Jackie reviewed and summarized numerical findings from quantitative and mixed-methods studies and generated several indicators to measure the effectiveness of multiple-choice tests. In phase 2, Jackie surveyed qualitative findings from qualitative and mixed-methods studies and used the numerical categories from phase 1 to explore them from the perspective of students, teachers, and school administrators. This provided her with a deeper understanding of the nuances involved in the efficacy of using multiple-choice tests to assess students' knowledge.

Convergent Synthesis

From the perspective of convergent synthesis design, qualitative, quantitative, and mixed-methods research studies can address the same questions and therefore do

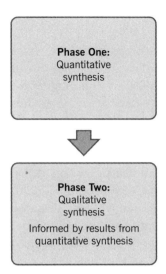

FIGURE 9.8. The process of sequential explanatory synthesis.

not require separate synthesis methods (Hannes, 2015). Thus, in this type of synthesis, research studies are grouped by findings rather than by design (Sandelowski et al., 2006). The emphasis is on transforming findings from qualitative, quantitative, and mixed-methods studies in order to combine and integrate all the results of the included studies. Thus, in qualitative synthesis design, the results from quantitative studies are transformed into qualitative findings, while in convergent quantitative synthesis design, qualitative results are transformed into variables. Figure 9.9 illustrates the process of convergent synthesis.

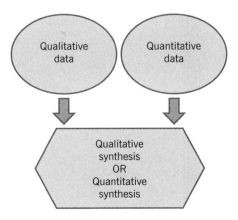

FIGURE 9.9. The process of convergent synthesis design.

Convergent Qualitative Design

This synthesis addresses questions such as *what?*, *why?*, and *how?* by using themes, concepts, and patterns to transform results from qualitative, quantitative, and mixed-methods studies into qualitative findings (Pluye & Hong, 2014). These themes, concepts, and patterns may be predefined, emerge from the data, or be a combination of both. Through constant comparison, the review writer uses a qualitative interpretive process and examines these themes, concepts, and patterns across studies, looking for similarities and differences. This synthesis method is mostly theory driven and allows the writer to build a line of argument and to assess a policy, an intervention, or a program.

An example of qualitative convergent design is a review for a dissertation carried out by Ronit, a student in public policy studies. She reviewed qualitative, quantitative, and mixed-methods research studies that were conducted on major standards-based reform efforts in the past two decades and the interaction between policy design and implementation. The review of findings from all the studies she has reviewed revealed repeating themes that may contribute to a theory on implementing educational policy reforms.

Convergent Quantitative Design

According to Pluye and Hong (2014), use of this design is still rare and may present a challenge to literature review writers. In this synthesis, results from qualitative, quantitative, and mixed-methods studies are transformed into numerical variables. This transformation is usually done through content analysis, where a large amount of textual data obtained through qualitative data collection strategies (such as interviews, observations, and documentations) is converted into defined variables. The results are then used for statistical analysis.

An example of a quantitative convergent design is a study by Antonio, who is working on the literature review section of his master's thesis in social work. He examined whether teenagers who try to kick their drug habits are more likely to be successful when they are surrounded by a supportive environment in comparison to those who are experiencing a punitive attitude by their family members and the school system. As part of his review, Antonio conducted a content analysis and identified several distinct categories that he converted into defined variables and analyzed statistically. He then used this information to compare the two approaches and assess the efficacy of each.

Your choice of the type of mixed-studies synthesis depends on your research question and the aim of your review. Make the choice carefully; these types of syntheses may present a challenge for reviewers who do not have knowledge of the theoretical and practical elements of both qualitative and quantitative synthesis. Throughout the process, be sure not to violate the different philosophical

TABLE 9.4. A Summary of Segregated, Sequential, and Convergent Synthesis of Mixed Studies

Design		Phase one	Phase two
Segregated synthesis		**Phase one**	**Phase two**
		Qualitative synthesis	Common conclusions
		Quantitative synthesis	
Sequential synthesis		**Phase one**	**Phase two**
	Sequential exploratory synthesis	Qualitative synthesis	Quantitative synthesis: informed by results from qualitative synthesis
	Sequential explanatory synthesis	Quantitative synthesis	Qualitative synthesis: informed by results from quantitative synthesis
Convergent synthesis		**Data source**	**Synthesis approach**
	Convergent qualitative	Results from qualitative, quantitative, and mixed-methods studies	Qualitative analysis
	Convergent quantitative	Results from qualitative, quantitative, and mixed-methods studies	Quantitative analysis

foundations of each approach. Use appropriate methods to bridge their differences and outline clearly, and in detail, the synthesis method that you have chosen for your review.

Table 9.4 summarizes the mixed-studies designs discussed in the chapter.

SYNTHESIS OF HERMENEUTIC–PHENOMENOLOGICAL LITERATURE

There are some similarities in the approach to synthesis of articles between the hermeneutic–phenomenological and qualitative studies. Still, hermeneutic–phenomenological literature review has distinct characteristics and calls for its own particular process of synthesis and interpretation (Laverty, 2003).

The central focus of this approach is discovering the meaning of a phenomenon or subject at the center of the review. The reviewer's role is not to "tell" the content of texts or to report objectively the ideas offered by their authors. Rather, literature review writers share the new insights that the original texts' authors have provoked within them (Smythe & Spence, 2012), and the review is seen as a conversation in which the authors and the reviewers become dialogical partners in a search for meaning.

In these conversations, reviewers do not silence their own interpretations or put aside their own perceptions. Rather, the meanings reviewers make of texts are derived from what Heidegger termed *pre-understanding* (Laverty, 2003), which refers to the reviewers' own history, culture, and life experience. Instead of silencing these pre-understandings, Gadamer (1998) suggests that reviewers should reflect on and disclose their particular world views and the philosophical vantage points that shape their syntheses and interpretations of the sources.

At the same time, reviewers should be open to the uniqueness of each source, allow texts to challenge and stretch their previous understandings, and think about their research topic in ways they may have not contemplated before (van Manen, 1990). Gadamer (1998) suggests that gaining an understanding in a dialogue does not mean merely putting ourselves forward and asserting our points of view, but rather allowing ourselves to be transformed and not remain what we were.

In this transformation, review writers reach a better understanding of the meaning of both the subject and the self. This meaning is always complex, multi-dimensional, and multilayered (van Manen, 1990) and rejects any simplistic guidelines. For this reason, reviewers who follow the hermeneutic–phenomenological tradition avoid the use of a fixed set of methods for synthesizing the literature. They view the term *method* as a rule-bound endeavor (Polkinghorne, 1983), whereas the synthesis of literature is a creative process that is "more a case of playing or dancing or rumination . . . rather than an application of methods" (Slattery, 2013, p. 137).

An example of a hermeneutic–phenomenological style of synthesis is a study conducted by Naomi, who wrote her master's thesis on the topic of the body image of teenage girls. In her literature review, she synthesized auto-ethnographical, narrative, and phenomenological studies, as well as poetry, literature, popular music, and the visual images in television commercials. She compared the different sources and looked for repeating themes among the academic research, the arts, and the popular media when it comes to how girls' physical and personality attributes are depicted. In writing her review synthesis, Naomi created a dialogue around the themes she had discovered between her personal perception of herself as a young teen and the sources discussing this issue.

While we recognize that synthesis in a hermeneutic–phenomenological study is indeed a free act of "seeing meaning" (van Manen, 1990, p. 79), we offer some suggestions often used by researchers who follow this approach that may help you in the synthesis and interpretation process. Additionally, although we describe the process in a structural, step-by-step manner, keep in mind that for hermeneutic–phenomenological writers, the synthesis of the sources is mostly a cyclical rather than a linear effort.

Primarily, when seeking to grasp the essential meaning of the subject reviewed, it is helpful to approach the phenomenon in terms of themes (van Manen, 1990). Themes in hermeneutic–phenomenological synthesis are the core aspect in the readings that illuminate the characteristics of the phenomenon and comprise its meaning. The analysis and synthesis of these themes is used to fuse the sources and reach a holistic understanding of the literature review (Patterson & Williams, 2002). This is a circular, inductive, and interpretive process; it requires a close reading of the texts, and being reflective, insightful, and sensitive to the language (Laverty, 2003).

Van Manen recommends three approaches for uncovering the thematic aspects of the phenomenon in the selected texts: (1) the *holistic* approach when the focus is on the overall meaning of the text and its fundamental significance; (2) the *selective* approach for a more in-depth reading with a focus on finding statements, phrases, or metaphors that capture the essence of the phenomenon being described; and (3) the *line-by-line* approach when single sentences or sentence clusters are explored in order to find what is revealed about the phenomenon or experience at the center of the review.

From the hermeneutic–phenomenological perspective, identifying and labeling themes and determining their meaning is an interpretive and creative endeavor that might be done differently by different reviewers. Multiple interpretations may coexist and no one interpretation is truer than another (van Manen, 1990).

TO DO: How to Create a Synthesis of Hermeneutic–Phenomenological Literature

Based on van Manen's description, we offer a set of flexible guidelines for thematic analysis and synthesis for your consideration in Table 9.5. You may want to creatively adapt these suggestions to fit the goals of your own literature review.

TABLE 9.5. Steps for Creating a Synthesis of Hermeneutic–Phenomenological Literature

Step
1. Identify emerging themes which seem to define the meaning of the phenomenon as described in the individual sources.
2. Separate the essential themes from the incidental themes and keep only those that distinguish the phenomenon and make it what it is.
3. Check and mark where the emerging themes appear in your source or sources and note commonalities among them.
4. Look for connections between themes and group them according to their unifying conceptual similarities; label each group in a way that captures its meaning.
5. Order the groups of themes according to the questions that guided your literature review and your own theoretical position. The final list should comprise major themes and subthemes.
6. Display the major themes and subthemes in a table or other organizational strategies.
7. Write an overall persuasive argument that reflects the interrelationships among the identified themes and offers a holistic meaning derived from their synthesized combination.

Figure 9.10 illustrates the major steps in searching, analyzing, and synthesizing themes using a hermeneutic–phenomenological process.

One of the fundamental concepts that characterizes hermeneutic–phenomenological synthesis is a constant dialectic movement between the whole and its parts. This movement entails understanding the literature as a whole, interpreting its individual parts, and then going back to the holistic understanding (Myers, 2004). Thus, when trying to gain an understanding of the trends that typify the topic as a whole, you should step back and evaluate the overall contexts of the individual studies. At the same time, the holistic understanding should be incorporated into the consideration of the meaning of each individual research

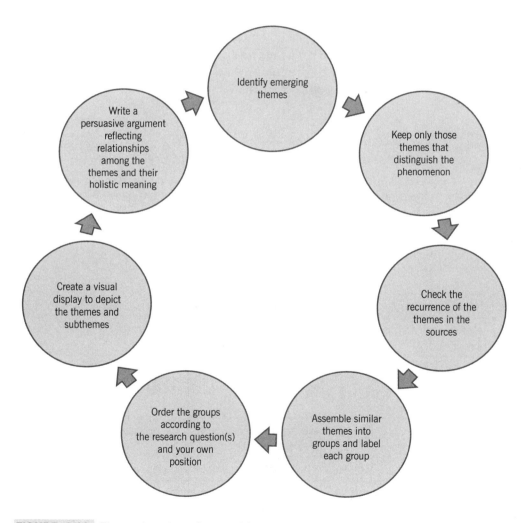

FIGURE 9.10. The major steps in searching, analyzing, and synthesizing themes using a hermeneutic–phenomenological process.

study. From this perspective, this constant movement is similar to the synthesis process of qualitative research.

However, unlike the process of qualitative synthesis, where the meanings the reviewer makes of the phenomenon are drawn mostly from that of the original researcher's interpretation, in hermeneutic–phenomenological synthesis the reviewer recovers the meanings through the eyes of the study's participants. At the same time, the review writer often steps back and sees the picture as a whole from a distance, finding the phenomenon's meanings beyond the original interpretation of the participants or the particular local context (Polkinghorne, 1983).

Gadamer (1983) called this constant dynamic movement of interpretation and meaning the *hermeneutic circle*. This circle involves the reviewer in a process of cyclical participation in reading, reflecting, and writing that leads to a new insight, defined by Heidegger (1995, p. 376) as a moment of vision, an *augenblick*. For hermeneutic–phenomenological scholars, this moment of insight is a "gifted grace" (Vanhoozer, Smith, & Bonson, 2006). Waiting for these moments of grace and unexpected understandings, while at the same time working intensively and seeking new insights, is "the interplay between seeking and waiting, of writing and pondering, of knowing and doubting" as "tentative understanding takes shape" (Smythe & Spence, 2012, p. 20). Figure 9.10 (p. 204) illustrates the major steps in searching, analyzing, and synthesizing themes using a hermeneutic–phenomenological process.

WHAT'S NEXT?

In this chapter we described the process of synthesizing and interpreting the traditional–narrative, quantitative, qualitative, mixed-methods, and hermeneutic–phenomenological sources for your literature review. In the next chapter our focus moves to discussing your role as the literature review writer and how you develop an authoritative voice.

CHAPTER SUMMARY

1. In a synthesis process, the writer weaves together elements from separate texts to create a new holistic story and cohesive argument. The two main forms of synthesis are *aggregative* and *interpretive*.

2. The synthesis in traditional–narrative reviews can be done by grouping sources, comparing and contrasting sources, exploring conflicting or contradicting findings, and adopting a critical stance. Throughout this process, be aware of your research question(s).

3. An essential requirement for conducting a quality synthesis of the literature on your topic is carrying it out with a critical stance.

4. *Meta-analysis* and *quantitative narrative* are two approaches used to synthesize quantitative sources to discover and explain relationships among variables and assess the internal and external validity of each study. Both approaches provide a systematic process that can be subjected to an audit.

5. *Meta-analysis* is used to analyze and synthesize numerical data from individual studies on the same topic or research question by combining statistical findings from multiple studies thereby yielding results that individual studies cannot offer.

6. *Quantitative narrative synthesis,* which is more intuitive, is a systematic review that summarizes and synthesizes results from multiple studies that include quantitative data using only words and text.

7. *Meta-ethnography* is an inductive and interpretative approach to synthesizing qualitative research findings and is the method most commonly used among qualitative researchers.

8. Three paths can be used to compare metaphors, concepts, and constructs among studies: *reciprocal*, *refutational,* and *line of argument.*

9. A synthesis of *mixed-studies* literature brings together quantitative, qualitative, and mixed-methods sources within a single literature review in a way that takes advantage of the strength of stories and the strength of numbers. There are four commonly used types of syntheses: *segregated synthesis, sequential exploratory synthesis, sequential explanatory synthesis,* and *convergent synthesis.*

10. The central focus of *hermeneutic–phenomenological synthesis* is discovering the meaning of a phenomenon or subject at the center of the review. It is done through three approaches: *holistic, selective,* and *line-by-line.*

CHAPTER 10

The Writer Voice and the Writing Process

At its heart, a literature review is a dialogical engagement with the writings done by other authors. Their ideas, theories, research, and conceptualizations stimulate your thinking and meaning-making. In your own writing, you seek to articulate your understanding of, and engagement with, the knowledge and insights gained from these authors' perspectives and communicate how your own thinking has deepened and evolved as a result of this.

Writing is a crucial and integral part of developing a literature review. Through it you communicate layered meanings and theories that you have constructed from existing knowledge, as well as the questions, tensions, and debates you have discovered. As you contemplate your own writing of the literature review, you probably wonder what your role as writer in this dialogical engagement is. Do you have the confidence to see yourself as a partner in a conversation with authorities in the field or do you perceive yourself as a vessel who merely transmits their ideas? Do you silence your own voice and express only the voices of the authors you draw from? Do you assert your presence in your narrative or step back, give up your authority as a writer, and foreground only the authors you review?

From Richardson's (1990) point of view, whether review writers admit it or not, or are aware of it or not, they use their authority in presenting the ideas of the authors they reference. Richardson states, "No matter how we stage the text, we [the literature review writers] are doing the staging" (p. 12). Still, you may wonder if there is room in academic writing for asserting your authorial presence. This decision is very important in shaping the style and stance of your review.

In this chapter we discuss the role you may want to adopt as the literature review writer and consider whether you want to use an active or passive voice. We offer different strategies for asserting your presence in your narrative and describe methods for keeping your ideas separate from those of the authors you review. We end the chapter by reflecting on how you might develop an authoritative voice and consider strategies that will allow you to overcome writing blocks.

PERSONAL PRESENCE IN THE LITERATURE REVIEW ||||||||||||||||||||||||||||||||||||||||||||||||||||||||||||||

As stated above, a literature review is a conversation among scholars. You enter the dialogue by articulating what "they say" and what "I say" (Graff & Birkenstein, 2014, p. xiii). Your ideas that were initially "born of another [author] or dynamically stimulated by another" will, in the process of your writing, liberate themselves from the authority of others' discourse (Bakhtin, 1981, p. 348).

As you enter this dialogue you make a transition from being a student to becoming a scholar and recognize your potential contribution to further the knowledge in your field. Being part of such a dialogue requires confidence in your ability "to identify the discoursal voice as well as your own voice and feel you have a right to speak" (Wisker, 2015, p. 65).

What is *voice*? Writer voice is the form or style through which the literature review story is told; it is "the writer's presence on the page" (Romano, 2004, p. 5). Foregrounding your voice refers to the way you present yourself in relation to the authors you cite and the audience you target (Ridley, 2012). Your writer voice reflects the way you bring together and incorporate the perspectives of the authors you review and your own viewpoints. Choosing the voice you will use is not a mere technique or writing method; your choice mirrors how you orient yourself as a writer toward knowledge and toward the literature you review.

In the past, academic writing was used to clearly define (and often impose) the relationship between the voice of the literature review writer and the cited authors. The traditional belief was that in scientific writing the personal presence of the reviewer should be deemphasized (Galvan & Galvan, 2017). From this perspective, in academic contexts, especially in science, engineering, and medicine, the reviewed studies are given a central role and are discussed from an objective point of view. The reviewer assumes a detached, impersonal, and passive voice to demonstrate that her or his presence has not affected the objective reporting of the source material.

However, in recent decades this convention has changed, especially in social studies, humanities, and education, but also in hard science writing. It is accepted that the reviewers' voices are brought to the fore as they assert their claims and express their points of view, perceptions, and stances (Ridley, 2012). Moreover, for qualitative and hermeneutic–phenomenological reviews the authorial presence of the writer is inherently essential (Wolcott, 2009). Recognizing the critical nature of the writers' subjective role in composing the literature reviews, it is expected that they will put their own personal stamp of authority on their review in relation to the source texts. They should adopt a "well-situated voice" (Elbow, 2000, p. 210) that positions itself in the conversation among the different authors of these texts.

Still, the issue of voice may be controversial in some fields, and some professors may prefer a traditional, detached, and formal style of review writing. Our suggestion is to pay attention to the conventions common in your discipline and to be sensitive to your audience's expectations. Consult with your supervisor, dissertation chair, or grant guidelines to determine what voice you should adopt. Keep in mind, though, the suggestion of Elbow (2000), one of the most influential teachers of writing, who claims that academic writers may use any voice they feel comfortable with when they write early, exploratory drafts. These drafts can always be revised and changed into the voice that their thesis, dissertation, or grant audiences demand.

First-Person Pronouns

Foregrounding your own voice while reviewing the literature can be done in a number of ways. The most obvious one is using singular first-person pronouns (*I*, *me*, *my*) and, in the case of more than one author, the plural pronoun (*we*, *us*, *ours*). At times (mostly in the qualitative and hermeneutic–phenomenological reviews), the pronoun *we* may also be used by an individual writer to bond with the readers and make them feel like partners exploring ideas together.

In the past, many writers, especially in systematic or quantitative reviews in the sciences, tended to avoid first person or used it sparingly and let the source material speak for itself (Danica, Ventura, & Verdaguer, 2013). From their perspective, using personal pronouns in scientific papers interfered with the impression of objectivity and impersonality that they felt was required in order to persuade the readers of the validity and credibility of their arguments (Galvan & Galvan, 2017). For that reason, they replaced the singular pronouns with the impersonal *the research* or used another noun as the subject of the narrative.

Conventions governing the use of personal pronouns have changed over the years. It is now commonly agreed by many researchers that the persuasion of an argument is grounded in the reasons and evidence the literature review writers provide rather than in their choice of a particular pronoun. Many academic writing experts and supervisors of dissertations and theses accept, or even encourage, the use of personal pronouns. The use of the pronoun is especially advised when, for example:

- ▶ Describing how you decided to choose your topic (e.g., "I chose this topic based on my experience as a social worker . . .").
- ▶ Explaining how you chose your sources (e.g., "I started with an online search of electronic databases . . .").

▶ Indicating the activities undertaken in writing the review (e.g., "I compared and contrasted research done on the topic of . . . ").

▶ Outlining how the review is organized (e.g., "I organized the review around four sections . . . ").

▶ Moving the narrative from one section to the next (e.g., "Based on what researchers have found, in the next section I focus on their application in the field . . . ").

▶ Asserting your views or assessment in relation to the cited sources (e.g., "In my view, this idea . . . ").

▶ Putting forward your claims or perspectives (e.g., "My argument on this issue builds on the claims presented so far and offers an additional element . . . ").

▶ Sharing your own professional or personal experience as it relates to the arguments presented by the cited authors (e.g., "The claim put forth by Johnson resonates with the experience I had while working in . . . ").

The advantage of using personal pronouns is that it enhances your authority and emphasizes your agency as a writer. This is especially useful when you highlight the original direction of your review and your own contribution to current knowledge. The use of personal pronouns also helps to distinguish between your presentation of the work of the authors you cite and your own points of view, thus avoiding vagueness and ambiguity. Additionally, use of personal pronouns adds energy and life to your writing (Elbow, 2000).

Nevertheless, using first-person pronouns excessively and having a series of "I" statements can be monotonous. Moreover, in some cases using first-person pronouns may be less effective. Phrases such as "I like," "I feel," "I think," or "It is our belief" serve no real purpose, since personal judgment cannot replace reasoned evidence or a reference to the literature. In short, as a writer it is important to take control of your narrative and use a variety of styles by moving between active and passive voices as appropriate (Hart, 1998). Table 10.1 compares the use of a personal active format and a passive format.

TABLE 10.1. Comparing the Use of Active and Passive Formats	
Active format	**Passive format**
For the purpose of my research **I adopted** van Manen's practice.	For the purpose of this research van Manen's practice **was adopted**.
I divided my discussion into three sections.	The discussion **was divided** into three sections.
Based on the evidence, **we concluded** that. . . .	The evidence **led to a conclusion** that. . . .

Another issue that you may wonder about is whether it is permitted to include personal experiences in your literature review. In systematic reviews and in any review that emphasizes the writer's objectivity, sharing personal experiences may not be welcomed. However, in traditional–narrative reviews that include mostly qualitative studies and, even more so, in hermeneutic–phenomenological reviews, incorporating personal or professional experiences in relation to your topic is accepted and even encouraged. Sharing your experiences can, for example, serve as a rationale for selecting an issue as a focus of your study, be part of your reflections on your subjectivity and biases, or demonstrate the practical meanings of the abstract concepts you discuss. However, reflection on personal experiences should never become an end in itself. Although the development of a reflective stance is one of the goals of thesis or dissertation writing (Douglas, 2014), these reflections should always be purposeful, relate to your analysis of the literature, and be used for persuading your readers to accept your claims.

In a word, the use of first-person pronouns and the inclusion of personal experiences depend largely on your field of study, your audience, and the field's stylistic conventions. We suggest considering the voice that feels most comfortable to you, looking into the academic publications in your discipline, or consulting your supervisor to determine how your purpose, audience, and natural writing style may be affected by the way you narrate your review (Elbow, 2000).

Establishing an Authorial Voice without Using Personal Pronouns

Whether or not you use first-person *I* or *we,* there are additional ways to assert your writer voice. Ridley (2012) outlines a range of strategies, some explicit and others more subtle. These strategies allow review writers to demonstrate their authorial voice and summarize texts in ways that advance their own research agenda. The following discussion delineates several of these strategies and provides examples to illustrate their use.

Unattributed Assertions Followed by Support from References

You may present a claim without using any citations and take ownership for its content. This assertion is then followed by one or more statements drawn from your selected sources that provide information to support, elaborate, or explain your claim. While you partner with the cited authors in stating a point, you are able to highlight your active role as a writer who controls the review's narrative. Our example in Box 10.1 (p. 212) is taken from an article that discusses interventions for refugees and war-traumatized youth (Sullivan & Simonson, 2016, p. 505). The first sentence states the author's claim, and the following sentences elaborate on the kinds of traumas experienced by the young refugees.

BOX 10.1. An Example of Uncited Opening Sentence Followed by Referenced Statements

Many factors may lead individuals to flee their home countries, but most refugees experience some level of trauma prior to flight. Refugees often experience significant psychological distress due to exposure to direct or indirect trauma, as well as intergenerational trauma transferred between family members (Baker & Shalhoub-Kevorkian, 1999).

Source: Sullivan and Simonson (2016).

Indicating Relationships among Citations

A subtle strategy for revealing your writer voice is to present logical transitions among the works of the cited authors. You want to stay away from introducing one source after another (such as: *X* says . . . , *Y* proposes . . . , *Z* claims . . .) without indicating the relationships among these authors' ideas. Without presenting to the reader how the references are connected to each other you allow the cited authors to dominate your narrative while you are kept passively hidden behind them. Instead, you want to demonstrate your authorial voice by presenting the work of the cited authors according to your interpretation of how they connect to each other and to your own claim. To achieve that, use words or phrases that indicate how the references are similar or different, or how they extend, explain, or challenge each other. Examples of connecting words you may use are: "on the other hand," "whereas," "in agreement with," "similarly," "furthermore," "regardless," "moreover," "While Naor (2017) states . . . ," "Thompson (2016) proposes that . . . ," or "building on Brown's position . . . "

BOX 10.2. Indication of Relationships among Citations

Gelven (1973) writes that an investigation seeks factual, scientific, and propositional knowledge, and once the guiding problem or question is "solved" or "answered" the study is terminated. . . . **Using Gelven's language**, an investigatory approach to educational phenomena characterizes contemporary educational research. This investigatory approach reveals a conception of education as a technique, as a science, and, ultimately, as a "numbers" game (Greene, 1987; Grundy, 1987; Pinar, 1995; Taubman, 2009; Magrini; 2014). **But** Grumet (1992) reminds us that . . . "Too often we flee," as educational researchers, "from ambiguity to mechanistic and analytic descriptions of the process of education" (p. 31). . . . **Moreover**, when education is reduced to mere numbers and categories, its ontological meaning is lost (Aoki, 2004; Taubman, 2009; Magrini; 2014). [Bold added for emphasis.]

Source: Dewar (2015).

The excerpt in Box 10.2 (p. 212) is taken from Matthew Dewar's (2015, p. 22) dissertation and presents the use of connecting words and transitional phrases (highlighted in bold) illuminate the logical connections between the ideas about educational research.

Using Evaluative Verbs, Adverbs, Adjectives, and Phrases

A useful way to foreground your voice as a writer is by interweaving verbs, adjectives, adverbs, and phrases within the narrative. These interwoven words hint subtly or explicitly at your view about the assertions or research findings conveyed by the authors whose work you reviewed. They may indicate your attitude regarding the cited authors' ideas—whether you support and praise or, alternatively, tentatively accept or critique their positions. Examples of such verbs, adverbs, adjectives, or phrases can be found in Table 10.2.

Writing an Overall Summary at the End of a Section or Chapter

Another effective strategy for foregrounding your presence is to summarize the main points offered by the citations discussed at the end of a section or a chapter. Such a summary is usually written when you want to highlight a point, a position, or an assertion offered in the cited sources. Avoid presenting a simple inventory list; rather, recap these ideas and connect them around your own central argument (Graff & Birkenstein, 2014). The summary is usually introduced by words such as "in sum," "to summarize," "in short," or "in conclusion."

For an example of such a summary, we can turn again to Dewar's (2015, pp. 113–114) dissertation. The excerpt in Box 10.3 (p. 214) comes at the end of a section where he discusses the etymological meanings of the words *education* and *well-being*.

TABLE 10.2. Examples of Evaluative Verbs, Adverbs, Adjectives, and Phrases

Verbs	Adverbs	Adjectives	Phrases
■ Agree/disagree with ■ Aware/not aware ■ Impressed by ■ Question ■ Doubt ■ Overlook ■ Object	■ Convincingly ■ Forcefully ■ Wholeheartedly ■ Consistently ■ Overly ■ Adversely ■ Unsubstantially	■ Salient ■ Appropriate ■ Significant ■ Important ■ Difficult ■ Questionable	■ There is no question that . . . ■ The assumption presented needs to be reexamined ■ The latest findings add weight to the claim that . . . ■ This seminal thinker illuminates an essential aspect . . . ■ A well-known and respected model describing the cognitive process . . . ■ The current theory is inadequate for addressing the . . . ■ The results of the study should be treated with caution because . . .

BOX 10.3. Overall Summary at the End of a Section or Chapter

In summary, *education* and *well-being* are descriptions of a process through which our potential for being is uncovered, nurtured, and expressed in more meaningful ways. Or in a more poetic sense, *education is the process of uncovering being from the well, the process of discovering and nurturing a more meaningful human way of being.* Therefore, a brief etymological exploration of what it means to be "human" might also help us better understand the meaning of education and well-being. [Emphasis in the original.]

Source: Dewar (2015).

Writing an Evaluative Summary at the End of a Section or Chapter

You may also use the summary to demonstrate your control of the references you use by incorporating evaluative comments into it. In this case, after summarizing the section or the chapter, you evaluate the ideas presented, indicating agreement or disagreement, praise or critique from the perspective of the argument you put forward in the review.

An example of an evaluative summary (see Box 10.4) is taken from a meta-analysis study by Lazonder and Harmsen (2016, p. 685) that synthesizes the results of 72 studies comparing the effectiveness of different types of inquiry-based learning. As the authors summarize previous reviews, they highlight the strengths of this method of instruction, and build their argument toward what needs to be further explored.

BOX 10.4. An Example of an Evaluative Summary

In conclusion, the research integrations presented in this section provide convincing guidance that inquiry-based methods can be more effective than other, more expository methods of instruction. Its effectiveness has mainly been demonstrated on learning outcomes assessed after the task by means of domain knowledge posttests; embedded assessment of the actions learners perform during an inquiry. . . . The second conclusion that can be drawn is that the effectiveness of inquiry learning depends almost entirely on the availability of appropriate guidance. . . . Finally, even though previous meta-analyses have paid attention to possible moderating effects due to the learners' age, the relative effectiveness of different types of guidance for different age groups has not yet been assessed.

Source: Lazonder and Harmsen (2016).

Selecting the Citation Patterns

Finally, you foreground your role as a writer by making a choice of citation pattern. Ridley (2012) distinguishes between two basic styles of citations, *nonintegral* and *integral*. Nonintegral citation allows you to emphasize the ideas more than the authors from whom these ideas were drawn. By comparison, an integral citation highlights the particular authors, whose theories, thoughts, or studies you have summarized.

Nonintegral Citations

The name of the author whose work you discuss appears in parentheses outside the structure of the sentence, as, for example, "Counselors provide services that support young adults in a myriad of ways, including attending to their social and emotional needs" (Klokovska, 2014). The advantage of such a style of referencing is that the readers' attention is focused around the information attributed to the cited authors rather than the authors involved. For that reason, such a pattern is also known as an information-prominent or research- prominent citation (Lynch, 2014).

Integral Citations

Conversely, when you use an integral citation pattern, the author of the source you are referencing appears as part of the structure of a sentence (Onwuegbuzie & Frels, 2016; Ridley, 2012). This pattern is commonly used when the writer wants to highlight the voice of the authors being cited by giving them a dominant role when their studies, ideas, theories, or conceptualization are reported. You may use this style of citation, also known as author-prominent citation (Lynch, 2014), when you are referencing prominent authors and researchers in your field.

Integral citation can take several forms. In the following list we provide examples of some of those that are most commonly used.

1. The cited author's name serves as the grammatical subject of the sentence that discusses the author's work. For example:

   Jackson and Meyer (2018) conceptualize good mentoring as responsive and supportive of their mentees' diverse social, cultural, and lingual backgrounds.

2. The cited author's name is an adjunct part of the sentence. For example:

   According to Jackson and Meyer (2018), quality mentoring constitutes responsiveness to and support for the mentees' diverse social, cultural, and lingual backgrounds.

3. The author's name is an agent of a passive sentence. For example:

> A conceptualization of quality mentoring was created by a responsive attitude and support toward mentees with diverse backgrounds, **as suggested by Jackson and Meyer (2018)**.

The author's name is part of a possessive noun form. For example:

> **Jackson and Meyer's (2018) conceptualization** of quality mentoring centers on being responsive and supportive of mentees' diverse social, cultural, and lingual backgrounds.

The strategies discussed above offer you different ways of foregrounding your authorial role and demonstrating your writer voice as you analyze and synthesize the work of the authors included in your review. It is no less important for you to differentiate between your voice and those of authors and make it clear when you move "from what *they* say to what *you* say without confusing readers about who is saying what" (Graff & Birkenstein, 2014, p. 68). This differentiation is the focus of the next section.

Differentiating between Your Ideas and Authors' Ideas

A literature review is, in many ways, a dialogue between you, the writer, and the authors whose ideas, positions, and studies you are reviewing. Lack of careful distinction between your voice and their voices leads to confusion for your readers, who may be uncertain whether you are expressing your own or someone else's ideas (Dawidowicz, 2010). You may even be accused, as Dawidowicz warns, of purposefully misrepresenting the source of your ideas in order to advance your own agenda. No less damaging to your credibility as a writer is that readers may accuse you of plagiarism (see Chapter 11), attempting to attribute the work of others to yourself. To avoid such confusion between your voice and that of authors, be sure to clearly separate your ideas from theirs.

The most obvious separation is using the first-person "I" or "we" as a clue to your reader that a particular statement should be attributed to you. The example in Box 10.5 (p. 217) is taken from April Jordan's (2015, p. 40) dissertation where she describes Charles Taylor and Maxine Greene's perception of narrative in order to justify her own use of narrative for studying educators who saw themselves as catalysts for social change.

Even when you prefer to limit or even avoid the use of first person in your literature review, you can signal to the readers when you are offering someone else's ideas and when you are presenting your own views. This can be done when you ensure that the citations are a way that makes it clear to whom a statement is attributed. Box 10.6 (p. 217) shows an example where the authorship of the ideas is unclear.

BOX 10.5. An Example of Differentiating between the Ideas of the Review Writer and the Cited Authors' Ideas

Both Charles Taylor (1989) and Maxine Greene (1995) see narrative as a quest for understanding our lives. Greene elaborates further by proposing that this quest is "for a better state of things for those we teach and for the world we all share" (p. 1). **In my view**, this speaks directly to social action and the educators' aim to improve society for all.

Source: Jordan (2015).

The text in Box 10.6 is phrased in a way that makes it unclear where Chernilo's interpretation of Habermas's work ends and where Fleming's critique begins. It is also confusing whether the writer inserted her own assessment of Habermas's theory or just summarized the point of view of other authors. The same section (in Box 10.7), with minor changes in the text, makes it clear who is saying what.

BOX 10.6. An Example of Text Where the Authorship of the Ideas Is Unclear

Habermas's (1990, 1993) principle of universalism emphasizes the idea of impartiality in moral and legal discourse. This principle means that every norm should be accepted by those potentially affected by it (Chernilo, 2013). This universalist orientation makes Habermas's work stand out in contemporary social theories. However, from a feminist perspective (e.g., Fleming. 1997), the principle of universalism is not sufficiently universal because it does not include a clear vision of gender equality.

BOX 10.7. The Text Shown in Box 10.6 with Modifications to Improve Clarity Regarding Authorship

Habermas's (1990, 1993) principle of universalism outlines the idea of impartiality. This principle of moral and legal discourse means that every norm should be accepted by those potentially affect by it (Chernilo, 2013). Such a universal orientation makes Habermas's work stand out in contemporary social theories. However, as Fleming (1997) asserts, from a feminist perspective, Habermas's principle of universalism is not sufficiently universal because it does not include a clear vision of gender equality.

GROUP WORK

1. Each member of the group should select a section from a draft of his or her literature review. Working as a group, identify the strategies that have been used to highlight the authorial voice and the presence of the writer. Consider whether this voice is adequately brought to the fore as the claims and arguments are presented. As a reminder, we are listing the strategies offered in this chapter. (Keep in mind that not all the strategies need to be used.)

   a. First-person pronoun
   b. Unattributed assertions followed by support from references
   c. Indicating relationships among citations
   d. Using evaluative verbs, adverbs, adjectives, phrases
   e. Writing an overall summary at the end of a section or chapter
   f. Writing an evaluative summary at the end of a section or chapter
   g. Selecting nonintegral and integral citation patterns

2. As a group, go over a draft of a literature review of one of the group's members. Check how the writer separated his or her voice from that of the cited author(s). In case this was not done properly, provide suggestions on how to rewrite those sections to make a distinction between the voices.

DEVELOPING AN AUTHORITATIVE VOICE AND THE PROCESS OF WRITING

Finding one's writing voice is not merely an issue of strategies and formal techniques. These are important; however, if you are focusing only on them, you are running the risk of diminishing the importance of your authoritative role as a writer. Lack of confidence is often reflected in your writing voice.

One of the challenges novice academic writers face is the transition from being students and consumers of knowledge to becoming knowledgeable producers in their role as literature review writers (Mays & Smith, 2009; Nolte, Bruce, & Becker, 2015). The shift often involves uncertainty and self-doubt about their ability to write as an authority when, in reality, they do not feel authoritative (Kalmer & Thomson, 2008; Wisker, 2012). Consequently, when they discuss ideas presented by leaders in their field, they often feel timid and apprehensive and tend to surrender their own voice to that of the authors they reference.

Bakhtin (1981) discusses the struggle encountered by novice writers as they seek their own voice while engaging with authorities in their subject areas. Voice, for Bakhtin, is the ownership of one's voice and ideas while addressing and responding to those of others (Cazden, 1993). Thus, to own their voice, beginning writers need to learn how to dialogue with other authors without being dominated by them. The words of others should be assimilated and reworked to serve the writers' own purposes, reinforce their own claims, and contribute to building their own arguments. When this is not done, Bakhtin (1981) warns, other people's ideas "exists in other people's mouths, in other people's contexts, serving other people's intentions" (pp. 293–294). Only when the reviewer takes these authors' work and "populates it with his own intention" do these ideas, inspired by the original authors, become their own. Or, as was stated by Bakhtin, "It is from there that one must make the word, and make it one's own."

Through reading, thinking, interpreting, writing, and rewriting, academic writers gradually develop confidence in their knowledge, independence, and ability to participate as equals in an academic discourse. This growth is expressed in their gradual development of an authoritative and dialogical voice.

In the remaining portion of this chapter we discuss the process of developing authoritative, authentic, and dialogical voice through the writing process. We examine the preliminary writing of the literature review drafts, consider factors that may inhibit one's writing, and offer strategies to overcome writing apprehension.

Preliminary Writing

At the early stages of the literature review journey you may feel that you lack the understanding and knowledge required for writing. Some dissertation and thesis writers may think that it is inappropriate to start writing before they are fully exposed to the full range of theories and studies on the issue at the center of their investigation. They prefer planning and thinking *about* the writing rather than actually sitting down and writing.

Wilcott (2009) repudiates this notion, saying, "You cannot begin writing early enough." (p. 18). The writer Lomask (1987) concurs, "Irrespective of where your research stands, start writing the minute some material begins coming together in your mind. . . . Get the words down. You can always change them." (pp. 26–27).

Most teachers of writing offer the same advice and recommend that you do not just think about writing but rather write. "Writing *is* thinking," they say (Wilcott, 2009, p. 18; Richardson & St. Pierre, 2005, p. 967); or as Douglas (2014) emphasizes, "Writing and thinking are extensions of each other" (p. 142). As we put our thoughts into words, van Manen (1990) suggests, we capture the internal and make it external, we verbalize our elusive ideas, and "come to know what we know" (p. 127). At times, we may even surprise ourselves when we discover unexpected ideas that are revealed to us in our narrative, or as Richardson and St. Pierre (2005, p. 967) acknowledge, "Writing *is* indeed a seductive and tangled *method* of discovery."

Early writing is not only a way of discovering what we already know tacitly or explicitly; it also allows us to be aware of what we *still need to know* and how to go about filling the gaps. However, you may wonder what you can write about at the early stage of the literature review when you are just beginning to generate ideas about your topic. The following are some suggestions that you may consider. (You may also want to revisit Chapter 3 for additional ideas.)

▶ Delve into your personal and professional story, your experiences, and positionality as related to your topic.

▶ Highlight the social, cultural, and political settings and circumstances that make exploring the topic so pertinent.

▶ Outline the argument you want to present and explore your perspective and subjective stance.

▶ Narrate a critical (real or imaginary) anecdote that illustrates and demonstrates some problematic aspects of the topic.

▶ Write a poem that beautifully captures the nuances of the situation you are focused on.

▶ Quote lines from literary, academic, or other texts that powerfully grab the reader's attention on a point that you want to highlight.

▶ Report on a newspaper article that addresses the issue you are exploring.

▶ Provide statistics that emphasize the urgency of the problem.

Like many others, you may find that the initial drafts you have written are unsatisfactory: the style is somewhat wooden, your voice is hesitant, and the ideas are not fully formed. But rest assured, you will return to these preliminary writings and use them as a springboard for more lucid and polished statements, enriched by the texts you read.

Developing a literature review is an iterative process that reflects the novice writer's intellectual journey (Douglas, 2015; Wisker, 2015). As you develop your review and revisit the earlier versions of your writing, you will generate new ideas and layers in your expanding knowledge and discovered insights. Reading, thinking, analyzing, and interpreting your work will often lead you to a higher conceptual level, or as Wisker calls it, "a conceptual threshold crossing" (2015, p. 64). Additionally, your voice will gradually become bolder and more authoritative. In short, the continuing iterative revisions and refinements of the initial drafts, will demonstrate your growing maturity as a scholar and your increasing confidence in your identity as an academic writer and a researcher.

If we gave the impression that once you begin articulating your ideas, the writing process proceeds smoothly and seamlessly in linear fashion until it is completed, this is not our intention. Nothing is further from the truth! The process of writing for a novice literature review writer is never easy or steady. It is a complex endeavor that has its ups and downs, good days and bad ones. There are times of excitement and stimulation, when you feel a dynamic fusion of creativity and clear thinking; the floodgate is open, ideas flow, and words seem to almost write themselves. On the other hand, writing can also be challenging and frustrating. In those times, you hit stumbling blocks and the writing goes excruciatingly slow, or even stops completely. You stare at a blank page and you feel a sense of blockage in your writing; words refuse to form, thoughts fail to crystalize, and ideas are jumbled.

You need to move through the blockage and proceed with your writing. There are factors that are considered inhibiting to the writing process and there are strategies that facilitate it. The following discussion addresses both.

Factors That Inhibit the Writing Process

Writing apprehension is defined as "a subjective complex of attitudinal, emotional, and behavioral interaction which reinforce each other" (Daly & Miller, 1975, p. 11). The term refers to a sense of anxiety that is associated with an interruption of the writing process and writer's block. Based on a study conducted by Boice in 1997, Goodson (2013, p. 19) reports on seven common reasons academic writers give for being stuck in the writing process:

1. Writing is too demanding and unpleasant.
2. It is acceptable to procrastinate and put off writing.
3. I am not in the right mood for writing.
4. There are other things that require my attention right now.
5. I am not impressed by what is published these days.
6. I am concerned with being criticized and feeling humiliated.
7. I can finish it all in one draft.

Douglas (2015) cites Johnson (1992), who highlighted four types of blocked writers: (1) the *internal critics*, who are worried that their writing is terrible and not ready to be shared with others; (2) the *saboteurs*, who think that their ideas should be perfectly formulated before they are written down; (3) the *procrastinators*, who believe that they are not ready yet, and that having a few more days, or weeks or months, will make the writing much easier; and finally (4) the *perfectionists*, who never feel that their writing is good enough.

Strategies That Facilitate the Writing Process

The negative attitude, writing anxiety, procrastination, and perfectionism that are associated with writing apprehension and writing blocks may act separately or in concert in interrupting the writing process (Douglas, 2015). Writing experts offer several strategies that may help you overcome and move beyond these inhibiting factors. These include creating an effective writing environment, freewriting, rewriting (revision and editing), and group feedback.

Creating an Effective Writing Environment

An effective writing process requires dedicating sustained time to working without interruption. Incorporating an additional commitment into your already busy schedule is probably very challenging. However, it is essential that you schedule a consistent routine where several times a week you are committed to working on your writing. During those blocks of time, writing is all that you do. Turn off your phone, avoid e-mails and social networking, and eliminate any distractions that may break your concentration. Ask your family members and friends to respect your need for solitude and allow you the time and space needed for your work.

Another basic requirement for effective writing habits is to create the right space for your work. It could be a room or a quiet corner in your home, your office at the end of a workday, or a quiet and remote spot in the library. The important thing is to create the most convenient environment that suits your mental energy and is conducive to your productivity.

Freewriting

Elbow, who pioneered the concept of freewriting, defines it as "simply private, nonstop writing" (2000, p. 85). This strategy, he suggests, is especially useful in helping novice writers develop habits of writing without hesitation and discover their authentic voice (Romano, 2004).

Freewriting entails writing without stopping for a set amount of time (for example, 10–15 minutes). During that time, you write on a particular aspect of your literature review that is on your mind. Make no corrections; don't think about spelling, grammar, or punctuation. Don't check citations, and don't search for forgotten information or missing words. Just move on! The goal is to continue the spontaneous flow and not worry about the quality of the writing.

After the allocated freewriting time, stop and read what you have written. Your text is probably unpredictable, crude, or even an incoherent mess. However, you may surprise yourself with brilliant insights and genuinely powerful phrases, sentences, or even complete paragraphs. In the next 15 minutes, see what should be saved and what should be eliminated. Rewrite the narrative; add, cut, and reorganize. Get rid of repetitions, add the appropriate citations, find the missing words or locate the forgotten information, and review spelling and language mechanics.

The principle behind the freewriting technique is separating the generating phase from the editing task (Goodson, 2013). These are two different activities. While text generating is based on creativity and intuitiveness, editing is analytical work that is focused on details. Our brain, suggests Goodson, does not perform effectively when tackling both of these tasks at the same time. Better and more productive results are yielded when these two activities are performed separately.

One of the major benefits of freewriting is that, especially for beginning writers, it diminishes the inner tensions and pressures associated with writing (Elbow, 2000). Freewriting allows students to overcome and silence the internal "editor" that scrutinizes their written work (Coffin et al., 2003). As a result, writers develop confidence and feel more comfortable taking risks and expressing ideas as they come to mind.

Another advantage of freewriting is its contribution to the development of the writer's voice. Bypassing the control of the "inner critic," the freewriting experience brings to the surface intuitive insights, feelings, and inner thoughts that reflect the writer's inner voice. This inner voice needs to be melded to academic expectations and become more measured and ordered (Shaw, 2010). Nevertheless, the experience of discovering the authentic voice still resonates in the revised sentences and adds energy and presence to the academic writing, a quality that is usually a challenge for novice writers. Additionally, the "discovery" of the authentic voice may also help beginning writers "*experience* [themselves] as writers in certain transformative ways" (Elbow, 2000, p. 88).

In contrast to the spontaneous, nonstop writing that distinguishes freewriting, there is another style of writing that is methodological and deliberate. Wolcott (2009) refers to writers who employ this style as "bleeders" (p. 23). These writers work very slowly, agonizing over each word, and carefully crafting each phrase and sentence. They often do not stop working until they complete the number of words or pages they set as their goal for that day. Often, the first drafts that they produce are well written and well structured.

Wolcott (2009) suggests that most writers move back and forth, depending on their moods and inclinations, between the freewriting and methodological styles of writing. As long as you are productive and continue to write, follow the approach that suits you best and that ensures that you work consistently and keep the momentum going. As Murray states, "Writing produces writing" (quoted in Douglas, 2015, p. 143).

What do you do when you hit a "stuck place" (Wisker & Savin-Baden, 2009, p. 1), when the words refuse to come and the writing grinds to a halt? Even on such days, when you are not very productive and your creative capacity seems to dry up, keep writing! Bypass the tasks that require creativity and articulating ideas and focus your attention on other aspects of the process, such as revising and editing portions of the text you have written before, or complete other activities that are more mechanical, such as updating the references list or formatting the paper.

Rewriting: Revision and Editing

Revising and editing are essential aspects of the recursive process of writing and rewriting. As stated forcefully by Elbow (1998), "trying to write it right the first time" is a "dangerous method" (p. 39). The literature review cannot be accomplished in one sitting; rather, it involves a constant revisiting, rewriting, and refining your work, from its initial iterations through recursive editing, until you arrive at the final crafted text. Through these recursive efforts, the quality of your works improves, your arguments crystalize, and the language becomes clearer and more eloquent.

It is often suggested that you distance yourself from the draft by setting it aside for a day or two before you focus on revising and editing it. After taking a break, you are likely to read the text with fresh eyes and see things that you have not noticed before. You may detect text flow issues and recognize ineffective wording, organizational problems, or mechanical mistakes that make your writing unclear and ineffective.

The rewriting process moves from revising to editing; from a broader "big picture" focus to a narrower, closer reading of the text:

REVISING

We use *revision* to refer to a holistic read of the text that identifies big problems and overall flaws. The revision process includes activities such as examining whether the text responds to the literature review questions you posed, checking whether the claims are substantiated and convincingly build up your argument, and paying attention to the structure of the piece to determine if it flows logically. You may notice that some of your ideas are not fully developed and you need to add a narrative to fill gaps in the text. Alternatively, you may find that some texts are redundant and removing a word, sentence, or even a whole paragraph will tighten up the text and contribute to its lucidity.

EDITING

Once you have sorted out the big picture, focus your attention on editing. In the editing phase you slow down and attend carefully and methodologically to details. You comb the text, line by line, looking for confusing or obscured phrasings, checking errors in sentence structure and grammar, identifying inconsistencies in formatting, and noting mistakes in referencing, writing style, spelling, and punctuation.

Many writers claim that reading aloud helps them identify mistakes and awkward expressions in their work that they may not have noticed when reading it silently. You can try reading aloud either to yourself or to others.

Group Feedback

Revising and editing your work on your own is a fruitful and irreplaceable part of the writing process. However, group feedback is also a crucial step in the recursive draft writing process. Composing a text requires outside readers who will recognize aspects of your work that you have become oblivious to (Douglas, 2014), as well as help you overcome problems that you cannot resolve on your own (Elbow & Belanoff, 1995).

Peers who, like you, are in the midst of writing the literature review, serve as the best external readers. Such peers provide a sounding board for each other's writing that "yields a combined effect greater than the sum of individual effects" (Goodson, 2013, p. 91). When members of the group meet to read and respond to each other's work, a sense of belonging, collaboration, and trust is formed (Nolte et al., 2014). The participating writers feel empowered to take risks and try out new ideas, trusting that they will be supported and guided by their peers. Goodson describes the synergy that is created as the group members read each other's work. They simultaneously feed off one another's comments and brainstorm ideas and suggestions that help the writers improve the current iteration of their work. As a result, the literature review authors may see their writing in a new light or find solutions to stumbling blocks and frustrating problems they have struggled with before.

Two additional advantages of group feedback are strengthening your self-assessment and accountability. Assessing your peers' work improves your awareness of problems with your own writing. Helping other members in the group revise their work contributes to your ability to better recognize what changes are needed in your own writing. Accountability is enhanced as the participants are motivated to make progress in their writing before each meeting, when they are expected to share it with their peers.

Still, the quality and the impact of reciprocal peer feedback depend on the atmosphere that prevails during the meetings and whether relationships of trust and support are formed among the group members. Often writers, especially novice ones, associate feedback with being negatively judged and thus dread the experience of sharing their work. Two contributing factors help overcome the stress and anxiety: (1) ensuring feedback is not judgmental (Elbow & Belanoff, 1995) and (2) getting *lots* of feedback on a regular basis from the same people (Goodson, 2013, p. 90).

It is best when you and your group members view feedback as supportive and helpful and not judgmental or insulting. When you believe that the suggestions are provided with good intentions and by people who care about you, you are open to listening and learning from them. On the other hand, a critical and evaluative tone leads to a defensive reaction and a refusal to consider the suggestions. Additionally, receiving lots of feedback leads to an increasing sense of comfort with the process. You gradually learn to focus on the benefits of having suggestions offered by peers rather than on your perceived vulnerability. This growing ease increases if you receive feedback on a regular basis from people you have learned to trust. For this reason we recommend that the group meet regularly for an extended period or even, if doable, throughout the entire literature review writing process.

TO DO:
How to Conduct Successful Group Meetings to Generate Effective Feedback

There are different strategies for conducting group meetings dedicated to providing feedback on each member's work (e.g., Coffin et al., 2003; Elbow & Belanoff, 1995; Goodson, 2013). You may find the steps in Table 10.3 useful in conducting such group meetings.

TABLE 10.3. Steps for Conducting Group Meetings to Generate Feedback	
Step	✓
1. At the first meeting, it is advisable that group members collaboratively agree on the routines and ground rules for the meetings. For example, should they decide how frequently the group will meet? How much time will be allotted for discussing each person's writing? How much time will be devoted to reading each other's work and how much time for feedback? Who will facilitate the meetings: the instructor or group members? You should also decide whether reading each other's work before the meetings is required or optional.	
2. After deciding on the meeting routines, in the meetings that follow, when it's your turn to share, begin by guiding the group members' attention to what you are looking for. Do you want the group to focus on a particular section of your literature review or do you want them to provide feedback on your writing as a whole? Do you want the group's help with sections in the text you are struggling to interpret?	
3. While group members provide feedback, do not get defensive or argue; rather, sit back and listen openly and carefully and take notes.	
4. After feedback has been offered, make sure you fully understand all the comments and suggestions. When there are conflicting suggestions, try to reconcile among them with help from the group.	
5. At the end of the meeting, your group members may write comments on the reviewed text and share them with you.	
6. After the meeting, consider what suggestions to accept and what to disregard, and revise your text accordingly. You, as the writer, are in charge of your work. The decisions you make as well as the consequences are all yours.	

Elbow and Belanoff (1995) distinguish between two kinds of feedback: *reader-based feedback* and *criterion-based feedback*. In reader-based feedback, group members express the experience they had as they read your writing and the impact it had on them. You may ask the readers to share with you what they felt while reading your work and how it affected them overall. Your fellow writers can help you discover whether your ideas are coming across clearly and provide you with suggestions on how to revise and improve your composition, brainstorming ideas on what can be added, expanded, or further clarified. This kind of feedback is especially helpful during the early phases of writing your literature review.

In criterion-based feedback, the group's response to your work is based on preset criteria. Group members can address specific criteria that you are concerned about or focus on specific troublesome features of your writing that should be modified to improve its quality. For example, readers' feedback can center on clarity, organization, your presence in the narrative and the authority of your voice, or the persuasiveness of your argument. While the group's focus should be mostly on the content and organization of your writing, you may also ask for help with the writing mechanics (e.g., format, spelling, grammar, and punctuation). Writing experts suggest that criterion-based feedback is most helpful for the middle and advanced phases of writing the literature review.

As you proceed with your literature review writing, you will find that both types of feedback are helpful. The choice of which will be most valuable at any particular group meeting depends on what suits your comfort level, your specific needs at that point, and what particular sections of the review you are working on at that time.

We hope that the strategies we discussed will allow you to overcome writing blocks, anxiety, and self-doubts and move beyond inhibiting factors to experience the joy of writing and attain a sense of accomplishment.

GROUP WORK

1. **Reflection.** Reflect on the literature review writing experience with your group members, discussing questions such as:
   - What aspects of the writing process did you find most rewarding and satisfying?
   - What elements of the writing process did you find most challenging and frustrating?
   - Do you feel like a writer? Explain.
   - What are some of the factors that may be inhibiting your writing? What can you do about it? What have you tried?
   - What strategies from those reviewed in this chapter might be most helpful for you at this time? Explain.

2. **Exercising freewriting**
   a. Set a timer for 10 minutes. Within that time, write quickly about a specific theme or specific ideas related to your literature review.
      - Write quickly and steadily, without stopping, until the end of the allotted time.
      - Don't worry about the quality of your writing, don't search for missing information, and don't check for mistakes or inappropriate wording.
   b. Set the timer for an additional 10 minutes. Within that time, slowly edit the piece of writing you just completed.
      - Eliminate any text that is meaningless or messy.
      - Look for repetitions of the same idea. When you find these repetitions, group them together and rewrite the text to eliminate the redundant sentences or words.
      - Reorganize the sentences logically and be sure that you use transitional words or phrases to enhance the flow.
      - Rewrite unclear phrasings, change words, and correct language mechanics.
      - Mark or note where you need to add more information, such as references and citations, definitions, data, or other material.

3. **Practicing group feedback**

a. Before the feedback process begins, decide on the ground rules as a group. Members may choose the kind of feedback they prefer: reader-based or criterion-based. The following questions may be used for each kind of feedback:

Reader-based feedback
- What crossed your mind when you were reading the text?
- What, from your perspective, were the main ideas of the text?
- Do you have suggestions for improving the clarity of these ideas?
- What specific aspects would you suggest that the writer work on while writing the next draft?

Criterion-based feedback
- How well is the text organized?
- Does the text flow coherently?
- Is the writer's voice clearly heard?
- Are there different points of view addressed?
- Are the claims backed by data?
- How effective is the language?
- What is still missing or what needs further elaboration?

b. Reflect on the process from your perspective as a person who provided and/or received feedback and share your thoughts with your group.

c. Consider ideas for improving the group feedback process that can be implemented at future meetings.

WHAT'S NEXT?

In this chapter we discussed your role as an authoritative literature review writer and considered strategies for enhancing the writing process and overcoming writing blocks. In the next chapter, we go over technical but required issues, such as writing styles, in-text citations, and reference lists. The issue of plagiarism is also highlighted in this chapter.

CHAPTER SUMMARY

1. Writer voice is the way you present yourself in relation to the authors you cite and the audience you target.

2. In the past, especially in science, engineering, and medical fields, the reviewer assumed a detached, impersonal, and passive voice; however, in the last few decades, the reviewers' voice has been brought to the fore not only in social studies, humanities, and education, but also in the hard sciences.

3. There are several strategies for asserting your authorial voice without using personal pronouns: (a) unattributed assertions followed by support from references; (b)

indicating relationships among citations; (c) using evaluative verbs, adverbs, adjectives, and phrases; (d) writing an overall summary at the end of a section or chapter; (e) writing an evaluative summary at the end of a section or chapter; and (f) selecting the citation patterns.

4. A literature review is a conversation among scholars, and you enter this dialogue by articulating what "they say" and what "I say."

5. To differentiate between your ideas and those of cited authors in order to avoid confusing readers you may use the first-person pronoun, and post the citations in a way that signals when you are offering someone else's ideas and when you are presenting your own views.

6. It is recommended that you start writing as early as possible. Early writing is a way of discovering not only what you already know but also what you still need to know.

7. Developing a literature review is an iterative process; through revision and refinement of your initial drafts you demonstrate your growing maturity as a scholar.

8. Several factors may inhibit the writing process, including a negative attitude, writing anxiety, procrastination, and perfectionism.

9. There are several strategies to facilitate the writing process, including creating an effective writing environment, freewriting, and rewriting, which consists of revision and editing.

10. Group feedback is a crucial step in the recursive draft-writing process because it can create synergy and help members brainstorm and find solutions to problems that inhibit their writing.

CHAPTER 11

Acknowledging Sources

Citations, Quotations, and Plagiarism

At this point, you have analyzed, interpreted, critiqued, synthesized, and organized the literature that you have read. Throughout the process you have been
diligently recording the references, citations, and quotations that you are planning on using in your literature review. In previous chapters, we offered different
ways of keeping track of your citations. Now that you are immersed in the writing
process, we address the issue of citing and crediting your sources according to rules
specified by the writing style that you are using. In this chapter we present three
leading writing styles; however, we focus on one of them to simplify our discussion.

Listing the sources where you found the information that you are presenting
is crucial. You should acknowledge the author of each reference you use in your
review and then again in a full list of sources at the end of the work. It is important
that you provide the full citations for all of the references that are listed in the text;
similarly, every work that you list as a reference must have been cited or quoted
at least once in your text. In case you are using direct quotations, include also the
page numbers where available (or paragraph number for online sources that do not
have page numbers). This places an important responsibility on you, as the author
of the literature review, and will ensure that you do not inadvertently plagiarize.
When in doubt, cite the source (Pan, 2008).

Your citations allow you to engage in a dialogue with existing researchers
and thinkers in your field and signal to the readers the points that you support
or oppose, and ideas that you want to expand and further explore. The following

summary of reasons for acknowledging sources is based partly on a list provided by the Purdue University Online Writing Lab (Driscoll & Brizee, 2015).

▶ Show your intellectual integrity.

▶ Add credibility and support to your argument.

▶ Show your respect toward the work of others.

▶ Recognize the researchers and thinkers who have influenced your work.

▶ Show how your review is based on previous work.

▶ Allow readers to expand their own reading list.

▶ Help readers find the same references that you found.

In this chapter, we discuss the issues of writing styles, citations, and plagiarism. We end the chapter with a brief discussion of the basic rules for creating a reference list.

WRITING STYLES

There are three major writing styles that are used by authors in a variety of disciplines. Whereas the exact format for text citations and referencing may change from one writing style to another, they all emphasize the need to properly credit and list sources.

The leading writing styles are (1) *APA style,* based on the *Publication Manual of the American Psychological Association* (American Psychological Association, 2010); (2) *MLA style,* based on the *MLA Handbook for Writers of Research Papers* (Modern Language Association, 2016); and (3) *Chicago style,* based on *The Chicago Manual of Style* (2017), published by the University of Chicago Press. APA style is the preferred choice for social science, sociology, business, and psychology, and it is also used extensively in education. MLA style is used in humanities fields, and Chicago Style is commonly used in history, sociology, and geography, as well as in the publishing industry.

There are additional writing styles used in other fields. For example, the American Medical Association (AMA) has its own citation style (*www.lib.jmu. edu/citation/amaguide.pdf*); and *The Bluebook: A Uniform System of Citation* (*www.legalbluebook.com*) is widely used as a citation guide in the U.S. legal system.

Before you embark on the task of writing your literature review, find out which writing style you are expected to use. If you are a student, check with your professor or your dissertation committee. It also behooves you to determine the style you should use if you are applying for a grant, or want to send your paper to a journal for publication, or to present at a conference.

Providing a comprehensive discussion of the proper way to use in-text citations and quotations using the three main writing styles is beyond the scope of this book. For detailed information about the rules for each of the three leading writing styles, consult their guidebooks.

IN-TEXT CITATIONS

In APA style and MLA style, referencing the works of others that you cite or quote is done in two places in your document: in the main body of the text and again in the reference list at the end of your writing (Ridley, 2012). Chicago style uses a different convention whereby the references are noted with footnotes or endnotes and the complete citations are listed at the bottom of the page or the end of the document, in addition to the bibliography at the end. For repeated sequential references, the convention of "ibid." (meaning "the same source") is used. An excellent resource for comparing APA, MLA, and Chicago styles is provided by the Purdue Online Writing Lab. This information can be accessed at *https://owl.english.purdue.edu/media/pdf/20110928111055_949.pdf*.

Next, we offer brief explanations and examples of in-text citations using APA, MLA, and Chicago styles.

▶ *APA style.* In this style, the author and date of publication are noted. For quotes, the page number is added as well. Box 11.1 shows examples of this style.

▶ *MLA style.* This style requires the listing of the author and the page number when citing a source. The page number is noted, without the word *page, p.,* or *pp.* The date of publication is not noted but can be found at the end of the document under "Works Cited." Box 11.2 (p. 233) shows an example of a text citation using this style.

BOX 11.1. Examples of In-Text Citation and Quotation Using APA Style

Example 1: In-text citation:

Reid (2014) asserted that the Pearson r correlation is the most widely used correlation.

Example 2: Quotation:

Reid (2014) stated that "when a statistical test is calculated to determine if a difference exists between two groups, with α set to .05, there is a 5% chance of rejecting the null hypothesis when, in fact, it is correct" (p. 289).

Source: Reid (2014).

> **BOX 11.2.** Examples of In-Text Citation and Quotation Using MLA Style
>
> **Example 1: In-text citation:**
>
> Embedded research is used in studies where both qualitative and quantitative data collection methods are used but one paradigm dominates the other (Efron and Ravid, 46).
>
> **Example 2: Quotation:**
>
> Efron and Ravid stated that "as a rule, quotations should be uses sparingly and only when they highlight essential points or are particularly well phrased" (29).
>
> ————
> *Source:* Efron and Ravid (2013).

▶ *Chicago style.* Using this style, the first time you cite a source, include all the relevant information about it, such as the author's full name, source title, and publication information (see Box 11.3, example 1). When citing the same source again, list only the author's last name, a short title, and page number (see Box 11.3). If citing the same source and page number consecutively, use the word *Ibid* (meaning "in the same place"). The references are noted in the text with sequential footnote numbers. Box 11.3 shows an example of Chicago style using excerpts from a term paper titled *Medical Innovation in the Civil War Era,* written by Lindsey Ravid (2015).

> **BOX 11.3.** An Example of In-Text Citations and Quotation Using Chicago Style
>
> Efforts were made to correct mistakes in "all matters relating to the comfort and health of the troops" and to try to create a safer and more hygienic hospital.[34] The rate of soldier deaths in hospitals slowly but surely declined after the hygiene system was implemented. For example, from October 1862 to November 1862 the mortality rate decreased month-over-month by approximately 23%, taking into account the total number of patients under treatment and the resulting fatalities in each of those months.[35] In addition, the numbers of soldiers catching diseases or contracting infections also fell.[36] The invention and implementation of sanitation standards in hospitals and other medical care centers saved many lives that would have been lost if the cleanliness regulations had not been enforced.
>
> ————
> [34]Chas. S. Tripler, "Report of Surg. Charles S. Tripler, Medical Director of the Army of the Potomac of the operations of the medical department of that Army from August 12, 1861, to March 17, 1862," *The Ohio State University.* Web. 24 Feb. 2015. Available at *https://ehistory.osu.edu/exhibitions/cwsurgeon/cwsurgeon/sanitation.*
> [35]Ibid.
> [36]Ibid.

As we mentioned above, we cannot offer an exhaustive description of in-text citations in this chapter. Therefore, we have chosen to highlight only the major rules and base our suggestions and examples on the widely used APA style. Make sure you modify this information if you are using a different documentation style.

Citations in APA Style

For any citation, only the name of the author and date of publication should be included. (For websites where no authors or dates are listed, include the URL.) This will provide the essential reference information without breaking the flow of the text.

When continuing to cite the same author in the same paragraph, there is no need to repeat the date of publication, unless the reference list includes more than one entry for the same author. When referring to the same work by the same author in subsequent paragraphs, list the author's name again. As to listing the date of publication again, it is often a judgment call or a style preference, so check what is expected of you. There are several ways to cite an author and you can vary and use them as you choose. The names of the authors can be noted at the beginning, the middle, or the end of the sentence (Ridley, 2012). Box 11.4 shows three citation examples: (1) the author is the subject of the sentence and the publication date is noted in parentheses, (2) the name of the author and date of publication are integrated into the sentence without the use of parentheses, and (3) the author is listed at the end of the sentence in parentheses, along with the date of publication.

If you summarize work from several different sources, it is often better to list the sources in parentheses rather than in the text in order to enhance the flow of your writing. In parentheses, alphabetize the works by the first author's surname followed by the date of the publication of each reference. Use semicolons to separate the different citations. An example is the following citation:

> Although a systematic review may include some qualitative research, most reviews of this type are quantitative and use statistical data (Gough, Oliver, & Thomas, 2012; Higgins & Green, 2008).

BOX 11.4. Examples of Different Options for Citing the Author's Name in the Text

Example 1: Johnson (2016) investigated the effects of. . . .

Example 2: The investigation conducted by Johnson in 2016 focused on the effect of. . . .

Example 3: The study was designed to investigate the effect of. . . . (Johnson, 2016).

When citing a work with two authors, both names should be listed every time you cite or quote that source. For works written by three to five authors, list all the names the first time you refer to this work, but in subsequent citations of the same work, list the first author, followed by "et al." and the date of publication (the words *et al.* mean "and others" in Latin). When a reference has six or more authors, list only the first author, followed by "et al." in the first and all subsequent citations.

In APA style, past-tense verbs should be used to report on research that has already been completed—for example: "Johnson **offered** several explanations for. . . . ;" or "Johnson **reported** similar findings. . . ." The use of present perfect tense (e.g., "Over the years, researchers **have found** . . .") is also appropriate at times, such as when discussing lines of inquiry conducted by several researchers (Ridley, 2012). It is also the right tense to use when reporting on research that started in the past and continues in the present.

Citing Primary and Secondary Sources

In writing your literature review, it is advisable to use primary rather than secondary sources (Efron & Ravid, 2013). As we discussed in Chapter 4, primary sources are reports written by the researchers who conducted the study, and secondary sources analyze and summarize research conducted by others.

When citing secondary sources, you have to make it clear to the reader that you are citing such sources and not the original ones. In APA style, the convention is to list the secondary source in the reference list at the end of the work. In the text, use the following convention:

Smith's study (as cited by Johnson, 2016) demonstrated that . . .

QUOTATIONS

Quotations refer to materials quoted verbatim from other sources. We suggest that you quote sparingly; quote only text that is uniquely phrased or beautifully illustrates the author's ideas and that you feel you cannot summarize or paraphrase. Do not overquote! Using your own words creates text with a consistent writing style (Feak & Swales, 2009), whereas using quotes excessively often breaks the flow of your essay.

It is also essential that you separate your opinions and conclusions from those reported by the authors whom you review (Dawidowicz, 2010). Your readers need to be able to tell whether you are conveying your own opinion or reporting information that was written by others.

It is important that you introduce your quotes and incorporate them smoothly into your text. In other words, quotes should not be left hanging as separate sentences. For example, if you are quoting text, you may use words such as those in Box 11.5 to incorporate the quote into your own writing.

If you quote lengthy copyrighted materials, including tables or figures, from another source, it is your responsibility to check whether permission is required for both print and electronic sources. There are specific guidelines for what is considered copyrighted material, which may vary among different copyright holders, so make sure you obtain the necessary permission if you use such materials.

The length of the quote may dictate how it is presented in the text. According to APA style, quotes of 39 or fewer words should be incorporated into the running text, with quotation marks. Quotes of 40 or more words should be typeset as an indented paragraph without the use of quotation marks. In each case, the author, date of publication, and page number are reported and the quote is introduced in the text. (See Box 11.6, p. 237.)

If there is a quote within a quote, it should be typed using single quotation marks. For example, in the quote from Efron and Ravid in Box 11.7 (p. 237), the words *yes* and *jumped* are typed in single quotation marks because they appeared in quotation marks in the original text.

When using a quote *cited* by another author, indicate the year of publication and the page number of the source you are reading rather than the quoted text. In the reference list, note only the source you actually read. In the example in Box 11.8 (p. 237), the review writer is citing Magrini, who, in turn, cited and quoted Gadamer.

If you omit text in the middle of the quote, use three ellipsis points (. . .) to indicate that material was omitted. You can change the first letter of the quote to fit your syntax (e.g., change from upper- to lowercase) (see Box 11.9, p. 238).

BOX 11.5. Examples of Incorporating Quotations into the Text

Example 1:

According to APA style (American Psychological Association, 2010), "The punctuation mark at the end of the sentence may be changed to fit the syntax" (p. 172).

Example 2:

An abstract, which is found at the beginning of the article, is described by APA style (American Psychological Association, 2010) as "a brief, comprehensive summary of the content of the article; it allows readers to survey the content of the article quickly" (p. 25).

Source: American Psychological Association (2010).

BOX 11.6. Examples of a Short Quote (39 or Fewer Words) and a Long Quote (40 or More Words)

A short quote:

Han and Love (2015) stated that "immigrant families are not all alike nor are their needs or interests" (p. 21).

A long quote:

Han and Love (2015) explained the reasons for a new model in order to better address the unique needs of immigrant families:

> To gain insights about parent involvement, many educators have turned to general parent involvement models that describe different ways parents interact with school. But these models do not adequately describe the unique factors affecting immigrant parents. A new model based on the experiences of U.S. immigrants from all over the world provides educators and community leaders with insights that help them tailor programs and services to support these families as they acclimate into U.S. school culture. (p. 22)

Source: Han and Love (2015).

BOX 11.7. An Example of Typing a Quote within a Quote

Efron and Ravid (2013) suggest that "respondents may be asked a question about a certain issue and if they respond 'Yes' they are automatically 'jumped' to another set of questions" (p. 109).

Source: Efron and Ravid (2013).

BOX 11.8. An Example of a Quote within a Quote

Gadamer (1992) highlights the contribution of contemporary fragmentation and departmentalization in higher education institutions to the sense of alienation that "occurs especially between student and student and between oneself and the society in which the students live" (as cited by Magrini, 2017, p. 171).

Source: Magrini (2017).

BOX 11.9. An Example of the Use of Ellipses to Indicate Omitted Materials in a Quote

Reid (2014) discusses the advantage of using the median instead of the mean in skewed distributions because "the median . . . is less affected by extreme scores" (p. 38).

Source: Reid (2014).

For digital publications where page numbers are not available, paragraph number should be included when possible. Note also that citations of articles in online journals often include an article number as well as page numbers, in addition to the volume and issue numbers.

When you take notes while reading different documents, make sure that your notes clearly indicate whether these are your own words or you are quoting from a source. If this is a quote, ensure that you have the complete identifying information because having to retrace your steps to find the citation information for a quote is very frustrating. (See Chapter 5 for our discussion of ANTICs.)

There are exceptions to the need to credit sources. You do not need to list sources or references for familiar proverbs or well-known quotations. Similarly, there is no need to list the source for information that is common knowledge (Menager-Beeley & Paulos, 2006) or a source that is in the common domain (Ridley, 2012). For example, the fact that Hawaii was the last state to join the Union (on Friday, August 21, 1959) is common knowledge and you do not need to quote the source where you read it.

CREATING A REFERENCE LIST

The writing style you use dictates how you organize and order the entries in your reference list or bibliography. The Purdue Online Writing Lab provides easily accessible examples of APA, MLA, and Chicago styles at *https://owl.english.purdue.edu/media/pdf/20110928111055_949.pdf*.

A complete explanation of the rules for composing reference lists is beyond the scope of this book. We encourage you to consult the guide for the writing style you are using to write your review. Here we highlight only some of the main guidelines for creating a reference list using APA style.

▶ List only works that were cited or quoted in your review.

▶ References are listed in alphabetical order by the first author's surname.

▶ For multiple entries by the same author(s), list chronologically, beginning with the earlier publication date(s).

▶ The components of each entry are authors (or editors), publication date, title, and publisher. For periodicals, note the title of the journal and other information such as volume and page numbers; for books, record the publisher information.

▶ For electronic sources, list the reference information, followed by the words "Retrieved from http:// . . . (listing the URL here)." When available, include the digital object identifier (doi) assigned by publishers to electronically available articles and other documents.

▶ Type the references using hanging indents (i.e., the second and subsequent lines of each reference entry are indented).

▶ Italicize the titles of books and journal volumes.

Word-processing programs such as Microsoft Word help in creating a reference list. In Word, this feature is available under the References tab. There are also free websites that you can use to accomplish this task (e.g., *www.citationmachine. net*). However, you should check each entry to ensure it follows the rules of your selected writing style.

After completing the list of references, check it against your in-text citations to ensure that they match. Sometimes when revisions are made to the literature review, references are added or removed and you need to update the list of references. A simple way to accomplish this sometimes tedious task is to use the "Find" feature in Word, listing the first author's last name and searching the document to ensure it was cited or quoted. Alternatively, you can go through the entire text searching every citation or quotation to ensure it is listed in the references.

GROUP WORK

Read the literature review of one of your study group members, noting the following:

1. Citations
   a. Are the references cited correctly in the text using the chosen writing style?
   b. Are all the references cited or quoted in the text listed at the end of the document? (You may want to place a check mark next to each reference listed at the end of the review when you find it in the text.)
2. Quotations
   a. Are the quotes in the text wisely selected?
   b. Are they well integrated into the text without breaking the flow?
   c. Are the quotes formatted correctly (for short and long quotes)?

3. Reference list
   a. Are all the entries in the references at the end of the document ordered correctly according to the chosen writing style?
   b. Are the references formatted correctly and do they include all of the necessary elements (such as author's name and publication information)?

PLAGIARISM

Plagiarism refers to using the work of others without crediting these sources. Such sources include both printed text and audiovisual media (*What Is Citation?*, n.d.). *Intentional* plagiarism happens when authors submit their writing knowingly presenting someone else's ideas or words as their own; *unintentional* plagiarism refers to carelessly or inadvertently quoting or using information from sources without crediting them.

The most glaring and obvious kind of plagiarism is the intentional inclusion of text from another source without acknowledging that source. The consequences for doing so are severe in academic settings as well as in public opinion. Less obvious but still with potential consequences are cases where ideas are taken from other sources without crediting those sources.

As the author of the literature review, it is your responsibility to know how to avoid plagiarism. Academic honesty policies are posted by universities and other organizations and associations (e.g., Council of Writing Program Administrators, 2003), and it would be a good idea for you to familiarize yourself with these rules. Helpful guides and student tutorials are also offered by many universities. Ignoring these rules can be a very serious matter and even cause the expulsion of an offending student from a university (Menager-Beeley & Paulos, 2006). When it comes to doctoral research, plagiarism disqualifies students' dissertations.

The easy availability of online information and full-text documents makes it easier to obtain and copy texts on every topic. At the same time, these online resources also make it easier to check for overquoting and possible plagiarism. One popular website designed to help students and instructors check submitted papers for potential plagiarism is the website Turnitin (*http://turnitin.com*).

Self-plagiarism can also be a problem. The APA publication manual (American Psychological Association, 2010) defines it as "the practice of presenting one's own previously published work as though it were new" (p. 170). Consider your previously published work as you would any other published texts and apply the same rules described in this chapter for citations and quotations.

How to Acknowledge and Cite Sources Used in Writing the Review

Table 11.1 is a checklist for acknowledging and citing sources in writing your review.

TABLE 11.1. A Summary of the Steps in Acknowledging Sources	
Step	✓
1. Use a chosen writing style consistently throughout the review.	
2. Credit each source cited or quoted, both in the text and in the list of references.	
3. Provide full information about each source following your chosen writing style.	
4. Clearly separate the facts you report from your opinion.	
5. When citing secondary sources, make it clear that you are citing such sources and not the original ones.	
6. Choose your quotations judicially and avoid overquoting.	
7. Introduce your quotes and incorporate them smoothly into your text.	
8. When quoting copyrighted materials, make sure you obtain the necessary permission.	
9. Avoid intentional and unintentional plagiarism.	
10. After completing the list of references, check it against your text to ensure that they match.	

WHAT'S NEXT?

This chapter describes the three leading writing styles, with a focus on APA style, as well as how to cite and create reference lists. The importance of avoiding plagiarism is emphasized. In our next and final chapter, we describe the key elements of a completed literature review and its interconnectedness with the other parts of your scholarly work, and offer assessment matrices to review your work.

CHAPTER SUMMARY

1. Most writing styles require that you list the authors' names and the dates of publication; for direct quotes, also include the page numbers where available.

2. APA style, MLA style, and Chicago style are the three leading writing styles; find out which style you are expected to use and follow it diligently.

3. Quote only text that you feel you cannot summarize or paraphrase adequately and ensure that you clearly separate the information you report from your own opinions.

4. It is important that you introduce your quotes and incorporate them smoothly into your text.

5. When quoting, cite the author, date of publication, and page number.

6. You do not need to list sources or references for familiar proverbs, well-known quotations, or information that is common knowledge.

7. Citing, quoting, or using sources without crediting these works is considered plagiarism whether it is done intentionally or unintentionally.

8. While the easy availability of online resources and full-text documents makes it easier to copy texts, these online resources also make it easier to check for overquoting and possible plagiarism.

9. To avoid self-plagiarism, consider your previously published work as you would any other published work and apply the same rules for citations and quotations.

10. After completing the list of references, check it against your text to ensure that they match.

CHAPTER 12

Putting It All Together

A literature review is both a *process* and a *product* (Ravitch & Riggan, 2017; Ridley, 2012). Most of this book focused on a discussion of the literature review as a process. We followed the different aspects involved in the non-linear and iterative process of writing the review. These include choosing a topic, searching for relevant literature, critically analyzing and organizing the chosen texts, synthesizing the material by identifying linkages and relationships among and across themes, and building a coherent argument that serves as a springboard for the proposed research. In this final chapter, we turn our attention to the written product that is the end result of this long and complex process. We describe the different components that form the literature review you are presenting to your audience. You have worked on those components throughout the process and now you are ready to pull it all together and construct the literature review as a whole.

Our discussion in this chapter begins with a description of the key elements included in the two parts of a thesis, dissertation, or grant proposal where the literature review has a major role: Chapter 1, the introduction; and Chapter 2, which is devoted to a review of the literature. We then explain the interconnectedness of the literature review with the other parts of your thesis, dissertation, or grant proposal. Next, we outline different formats for organizing dissertations and theses and how different literature review patterns are presented in each of them. This is followed by a description of different strategies that can be used to enhance the cohesiveness and flow of your writing. We end the chapter with suggestions for reviewing and assessing your complete literature review using assessment matrices.

REVIEWING THE LITERATURE IN CHAPTERS 1 AND 2 |||||||||||||||||||||||||||||||||||||||||||||||||||||||||

There is no single model for integrating the literature review into your dissertation, thesis, or grant proposal, and different academic communities follow different formats. For example, in most disciplines, the literature review appears in two separate chapters: Chapter 1, the introduction, and Chapter 2, the literature review. On the other hand, in the fields of medicine and the sciences, the literature review section is typically included in the introduction chapter alone.

There is also a difference between writing systematic reviews and most other types of reviews. While writers of systematic reviews are expected to adhere strictly to a given structure and preset criteria, writers of most other types of reviews have flexibility in how they structure their discussions, even though they are expected to include key elements in the review.

In this chapter we discuss the type of literature review format that is presented in two chapters: Chapter 1, where you introduce the readers to your work; and Chapter 2, where you critically review the literature on your research topic. In our discussion, we focus on delineating the common characteristics of all types of reviews while also pointing out aspects unique to specific types.

Our recommendations in this chapter are not intended and should not be perceived as a required template for you to follow. Rather, we are describing elements that are typically included in traditional theses, dissertations, and grant proposals. These components should not curb your creativity but rather serve as a general framework for you to consider. Make your own choices of the elements you want to include in your final draft and the order in which you present them. These decisions should be based on your research topic and on what is accepted and expected in your area of study. Additionally, you may want to examine the overall structure of the first two chapters in dissertations, theses, or grant proposals in your discipline, as well as consulting with the chair of your committee to help you make your decisions.

Furthermore, in this chapter we often refer you to more detailed discussions, guidelines, and suggestions found in previous chapters of this book. We suggest that you revisit these chapters, which outline the lengthy and intricate process of developing the literature review, as you work on the final draft of your review—the product of this process.

Chapter 1: Introduction

The introduction chapter is the reader's first exposure to your thesis, dissertation, or grant proposal. It should be engaging and pique the reader's interest in your work. It is also the initial foray into the intellectual conversation with your audience about your topic and should present readers with a clear overview of your study's landscape. It should clearly lay out the essential information needed to understand your study's goals and significance, outline the foundations of your own research, and make clear its importance and potential contributions to your field.

In the following sections we provide a range of components commonly included in the introduction. As stated before, the elements and the order in which you present them should be based on your specific research focus. Whereas the process of developing these elements is described in detail in Chapter 3, here we outline each of them briefly. These components are:

▶ Interesting opening

▶ Problem or topic statement

▶ Statement of purpose

▶ Definition of key concepts or terms

▶ Contemporary, theoretical, and/or historical contexts

▶ Significance of the study

▶ Research question(s)

▶ Scope of the study

▶ Road map of the study

Interesting Opening

You may want to open your introduction with an interesting "hook" that will grab readers' attention, invoke their curiosity, and encourage them to continue reading. This opening should be clearly and explicitly connected to the topic at the center of your work. It should capture the essence of your subject and foreshadow your study's importance.

These are some examples of what may be included in the opening to the introduction chapter:

▶ A powerful quotation

▶ Striking facts (backed by evidence)

▶ A set of relevant and referenced statistics

▶ A factual or imaginary anecdote or scenario

▶ A poem or other literary excerpt

▶ A passage from a newspaper or other media source

Problem or Topic Statement

State the problem or topic of your study early in your introduction chapter. The statement should be short and concise and clearly and unambiguously articulate the focus of your research; your readers should have no doubt about the issue at the center of your investigation. For example, you may state:

▶ "The problem I explore in this dissertation is . . ."
▶ "The focus of this study is . . ."
▶ "At the center of this research is the issue of . . ."

An example of a problem statement can be found in Jordan's (2015) dissertation study (Box 12.1).

Purpose Statement

The purpose statement, which often follows the problem statement, outlines the objectives of your study and what you intend to accomplish. It should be short (no more than three to four sentences), clear, succinct, and practical. You should make sure there is a clear connection between the problem and the purpose statements, and together they should influence and funnel into your research question, literature review, and research design.

In your purpose statement, you may include the research approach you are using in your inquiry and, when appropriate, add the target population and the location of the study. (However, it is not recommended that detailed design information and research techniques be offered in this section.)

To ensure that the readers have no doubt about your goals for the study, introduce it explicitly. For example:

▶ "The purpose of my dissertation research is . . ."
▶ "This thesis work is designed to . . ."
▶ "My goal in exploring the topic is to . . ."

BOX 12.1. A Problem Statement

The topic at the center of this study is the transformation that female educators are going through by engaging in social change and how such transformation impacts their perceptions of self and the world.

Source: Jordan (2015).

BOX 12.2. A Purpose Statement

The purpose of this case study is to explore the organization and management of a community-driven string music program under the direction of a parent-run board. This is a descriptive single case study that is focused on a public school, kindergarten through eighth grade, located in a middle- to upper-class suburb in a metropolitan area in the Midwest.

Source: Sarasin (2017).

Box 12.2 presents the purpose statement written by Karen Sarasin (2017, p. 4) for her doctoral dissertation proposal.

Definition of Key Concepts or Terms

You need to define the key terms and main concepts mentioned in your problem or purpose statements that are at the center of your work. These definitions help to ensure that there will be no misinterpretations of how these terms and concepts are used in your study. For example, when using the term *motivation* in the context of investigating people's behavior, you want to make clear whether you are referring to *extrinsic* motivation, which involves behaving in a particular way to earn external rewards or avoid punishment, or to *intrinsic* motivation, which is driven by internal rewards and interests.

To make sure that the precise meaning is not lost, you may want to cite authoritative references in your field, and even quote the definitions they are offering (Pan, 2013). For example, Sarasin (2017) has to define for the reader what she means by the term *community driven-program*. She has chosen the quotation from Issel (2014) shown in Box 12.3.

When there are disagreements or controversies within the academic field regarding the definition of a particular concept or term, discuss openly the

BOX 12.3. Using a Precise Definition from an Expert in the Field

For this study I am using Issel's (2014, p. 118) crisp definition of community-driven program. While Issel uses this definition for describing health programs, it reflects the phenomenon I am describing in my research: "A community-driven program has its genesis—that is, its design and implementation—in the involvement, persistence, and passion of key representatives or members from the community."

Source: Sarasin (2017).

ambiguities and variant meanings, and the different perspectives these meanings represent. For example you may state the following:

> There are critical variations in the way the term _____ has been defined and little consensus exists regarding its definition. The reason for the complex and variant understandings of the term is a disagreement as to its implications for practice. In my research, I use the following definition offered by. . . .

Contemporary, Theoretical and/or Historical Contexts

In the introduction, you want to contextualize your research topic by providing an overview of the contemporary, theoretical, and/or historical issues surrounding it. The contextual discussion may focus on contemporary issues related to current circumstances surrounding your research problem. It may include political debates, social hardships, practical challenges, or major conversations related to the issue at the center of your work.

You may choose to ground the contextual discussion around major theories, perspectives, or philosophical approaches underpinning the focus of your research. Provide a brief description of the theoretical framework that has informed your own approach and identify its major proponents and opponents. You may clarify the main principles of your chosen theoretical framework, its seminal trends, and research directions that are relevant to your own study. When discussing these theories or philosophies, it is recommended that you cite original primary sources of seminal writings rather than use only secondhand descriptions. (See Chapter 4 for a more comprehensive discussion of primary and secondary sources.)

You may also present a historical overview of your topic, highlighting its legal, theoretical, or methodological evolution over the years. In your discussion, you may point out landmark laws, seminal studies, or discoveries that have changed the way the subject has been perceived over time.

In the literature review chapter, you may discuss the contextual factors in much more depth, with additional, more comprehensive details. Additionally, you may choose to focus on particular contextual element(s) in the introduction chapter while discussing the others in the literature review chapter. It is entirely your decision which contextual factors should be presented in the introduction and which should be discussed in the literature review chapter. For example, you may decide to discuss the contemporary context in detail in the first chapter, briefly explaining the theoretical framework surrounding the topic, and then provide a detailed historical discussion and in-depth review of the philosophical and theoretical foundations of your topic in the literature review chapter.

It is important that the background discussion flow from, and be directly related to, your problem or topic statement. Make the link explicit and clear. Additionally, avoid presenting vague or overgeneralized assertions and be sure that your background information, claims, and propositions are supported by citations. For example, do not state something such as "Most Americans reveal a lack of knowledge of world geography" without having research evidence to back this claim. Similarly, avoid statements like "In the past, immigrants to the United States have faced legal hurdles and social challenges from official authorities" without providing a specific time frame supported by reliable references.

Significance of the Study

The discussion of the significance of the study explains why you have chosen to explore your particular topic or problem. The justification of your choice may include two parts: personal significance and significance to the field.

PERSONAL SIGNIFICANCE

Here you reflect on the meaning of the topic from a personal perspective. You may share what led you to engage in this particular research and share the positionality, ideological commitments, values, beliefs, and passions that have driven you to explore the subject. Some writers like to comment on the autobiographical origins of their interest in the topic and its roots in their life story or professional experiences.

This section may be a long, reflexive narrative or a short conceptualization of your personal connection to the research problem. In both cases, it is important that your personal contemplation be directly related and relevant to your research topic rather that a general account of your life story. Additionally, you want to reveal to readers your awareness of your explicit and implicit connections to the topic. For example, you may reflect on how your personal and professional experiences have shaped your frame of reference, underlined your subjectivity and biases, and formed your presumptions and assumptions.

The personal significance section is essential for those who write from the perspective of qualitative research or do a hermeneutical–phenomenological literature review, but optional for other approaches to the literature review. For systematic review writers, where objectivity of the researcher is emphasized, these personal reflections are viewed as unnecessary and unwelcomed.

SIGNIFICANCE FOR THE FIELD

It is essential that you discuss the significance of the study beyond your personal world and point to its importance for the field and for a wider audience. You want to highlight the study's contributions to your discipline and its benefits for particular population groups and organizations, or for society at large. The goal of this section is to convince your readers that the problem you have identified for your

research is valuable and should be explored. In your narrative, indicate the important contribution of your investigation and the potential negative consequences if
the current problematic situation is not addressed.

The significance of your study may be conveyed in its theoretical contribution
to the field, its relevancy to policy issues, its practical solution to a current practice,
or its focus on resolution through actions to address social justice concerns. Your
study may be significant for some or all or most of these four aspects, but mostly
the emphasis is on one in particular. Whatever your choice may be, make sure
you do not base it only on your personal opinion but rather add credence to your
claims by supporting them with evidence and citations.

You may also consider who your audience is and who will benefit from the
knowledge gained through your research. For example, is your audience made of
scholars? Practitioners? Parents? Policymakers? Academic or professional organizations? The particular audience you address in your writing will influence the
way you discuss the significance of your work. (See Chapter 3 for a more comprehensive discussion of the significance of the study and the study's audience.)

Research Question

The research question is very important in helping to ensure that your thesis, dissertation, or grant proposal has a clear and consistent focus. Your question should
be derived from your problem statement and should indicate the information that
is needed in order to achieve your stated research purpose. However, in contrast
to the problem and purpose statements that are more generally articulated, your
research questions should be more specific and focused. They should address
significant and important issues in your field, and should be clearly articulated,
answerable, and ethical. Additionally, in studies that lean toward a qualitative
approach the question is open-ended, usually based on *how* or *why* questions and
never elicit *yes* or *no* answers. (We discuss research questions in systematic reviews
later in this section.)

Typically, one to five research questions are presented, though three is often
the recommended number of questions. You may present a broad and general
"grand tour" question which is then broken into two to four more specific ones.
Make sure that you address each of these questions in your study, and have them
echo throughout your work. These questions impact your literature review discussion, shape the design of your research, and influence the strategies you use for
your data collection, analysis, and interpretation. Finally, the discussion of your
findings and conclusions should directly relate to your research questions.

In studies that are leaning toward a qualitative approach, the research questions may be refined and rewritten after you review the literature and become more
knowledgeable and insightful about your topic. Moreover, you may even reshape
and refocus the questions as you begin collecting and analyzing your data.

In systematic reviews, the research question is designed to assess and measure the outcomes and effects of an intervention, practical practice, program, or policy. It should be restricted in scope and clearly identify what is to be investigated, measured, and analyzed. Statistical analyses are used to test the study's hypotheses and to draw conclusions.

Scope

In this section, you outline the scope of the study, its extent, and its boundaries. You describe both what is and is not included in your research. For example, you may indicate that the study involves only female students over the age of 17 who are children of single mothers. Or you may indicate that your study is focused only on the stages of mourning rather than on all facets involved in the painful process of losing a family member.

Road Map

In this final section of the introduction chapter, you describe clearly, briefly, and concisely the topics you are going to discuss in the following chapters and thus provide a road map of your work. This roadmap enables readers to understand what is included in your work and how to navigate their way through your study. In the proposal stage, the road map is written using future tense while in the final research report past tense is used. Box 12.4 provides an illustration of a proposal roadmap.

Table 12.1 (p. 252) presents a summary of the components that you may include in the introduction chapter (Chapter 1).

Chapter 2: Literature Review

The review of the literature is written in the form of an essay. It is based on, and logically responds to, the research problem and purpose statements you have presented in Chapter 1. The literature review forms the scholarly foundations and

---

BOX 12.4. An Illustration of a Proposal Road Map

This topic of _____ was introduced in Chapter 1 of my dissertation and is further discussed in the following chapters. In Chapter 2, I review the literature and focus on the theory of _____. . . . . Additionally, I critically review studies conducted by prominent researchers in the field. This theoretical and empirical discussion leads to Chapter 3, where I outline my research paradigm and the research design that will guide my study.

TABLE 12.1. An Outline of the Major Components in Chapter 1 (the Introduction Chapter)

Components included in the introduction	Description
Interesting opening	Grab readers' attention and encourage them to continue reading.
Problem or topic statement	Present a concise problem or topic statement that articulates the focus of your research.
Purpose statement	Present a clear statement that outlines the objectives of your study and what you intend to accomplish. You may include the research approach, the target population, and the location of the study.
Definition of key concepts or terms	Define the key terms and main concepts mentioned in your problem or purpose statements.
Contemporary, theoretical, and/or historical contexts	Contextualize your research topic by providing an overview of the contemporary, theoretical, and/or historical issues surrounding it.
Significance of the study	Explain why you have chosen to explore your particular topic or problem. Your justification may include two parts: personal significance and significance to the field.
Research question	Articulate a clear and focused research question derived from the problem and purpose statements that will guide your study and its different components.
Scope	Outline the scope of the study, its extent, and its boundaries.
Road map	Describe the topics you are going to discuss in the following chapters.

framework of your own investigation. It is often the longest chapter in the dissertation or thesis.

In its essence, your literature review is a conversation with theoreticians and researchers about established theories and empirical work surrounding your topic. This conversation allows you to situate your study within the existing intellectual milieu and its traditions of inquiry. It also allows you to demonstrate your thorough knowledge of the field, build a strong theoretical foundation for your own study, and logically lead to your own research question.

While the review of literature draws on the work of others, your discussion should not merely mirror current knowledge but rather synthesize it through your own fresh perspective. You want your review to demonstrate generativity (Schulman, 1999); that is, establish your ability to learn from those who came before you. At the same time, you want to interject your own active voice as a critical interlocutor and expand and advance the collective knowledge and understanding of your subject (Boote & Beile, 2005; Ravitch & Riggan, 2017). (See Chapters 1 and 10 for a more comprehensive discussion on the literature review's goals, generativity, and contributions to the field.)

As we noted before, there is no single way of formatting the literature review and different writers have chosen various approaches, organizational structures, and formats. Throughout the book we have highlighted the impact of the choice of approaches to research (quantitative, qualitative, and mixed-methods) and their influence on the types of review the writer chooses (systematic, traditional–narrative, or hermeneutic–phenomenological). Although each type of review is distinguished by its characteristics, overall they share many common features.

Here we briefly highlight a range of different options that you may consider when you are writing your own literature review. Our description here is divided into the three parts included in the review: The introduction to the chapter, the main body, and the summary and discussion.

Introduction to the Chapter

In this section, you present a brief statement on what you intend to achieve in your literature review and how it is organized, including its major themes. You may also want to indicate the type of literature review you have chosen to write (systematic, traditional–narrative, or hermeneutic–phenomenological).

In systematic reviews, it is expected that writers describe in detail how the literature search was conducted and which keywords, databases, and other parameters were used (see Chapter 4). You also need to provide information about your criteria for inclusion and exclusion of sources. While this information is required in systematic reviews, there is a growing expectation that the process of source selection be transparent in other types of literature reviews as well (see Chapter 5).

For qualitative researchers writing traditional–narrative or hermeneutic–phenomenological types of literature reviews, the transparency may be expressed in the writers' reflection upon their selection of sources. They may contemplate how their personal biases about the topic of their research may affect their choice of references and their review of these sources.

The Main Body of the Literature Review Chapter

Our discussion of the literature review's main body is divided into four parts: (1) content of the review, (2) effective organization, (3) persuasive proposed argument, and (4) coherent synthesis and interpretation of sources.

CONTENT OF THE MAIN BODY OF THE CHAPTER

Various issues may be discussed in the main body of the literature review. These issues are framed by the problem statement, depend on the nature of your research, and logically link to the research questions you presented in Chapter 1.

As stated throughout the book, your review should provide the necessary background on your subject so readers can understand the nuanced contexts of the topic; the review should also logically lead to your study and shape the way you design it. Among the common themes often included in the review of the literature are: (1) historical background, (2) theoretical frameworks, and (3) methodological choices and past research findings. (See Chapter 5.)

Historical Framework. You may describe the historical origins of your subject of interest. For example, the evolution of a policy, a social trend, or relevant legislations and laws. You may provide a chronological account of ideas or concepts at the center of the topic as they evolved from earlier studies to current research. You may also follow major works conducted in that area, starting from seminal studies that became a breakthrough in the field, tracing how subsequent research has built on or criticized these major crossroads in your research.

Theoretical Framework. Another focus of the literature review may be the theoretical perspectives that underlie your work. You may present a school of thought or philosophy through which the phenomenon at the center of your study is viewed (e.g., postpositivism, reconstructionism, critical race theory, feminism). Or you may present an accepted scientific theory (such as Bandura's social learning theory [Bandura, 1977] or Bronfenbrenner's ecological system theory [Bronfenbrenner, 1979]) that presents general principles to explain the phenomenon you are researching.

Another option is to start by acknowledging and fully presenting the major theories relevant to your topic, including those you are critical of, before you zero in on the particular theory that you advocate. In your discussion, you should review the different facets of that theory. You may even put forth an argument that advances what is currently accepted in your field.

Methodology and Past Research Findings. Key approaches used for researching your topic and its disciplinary or philosophical origins may be another focus of your review. You may survey the range of methodologies and research instruments that have been employed in your field and highlight their advantages and disadvantages with regard to the investigation of your own topic of interest. Here you may critically analyze the merits and limits, strengths and weaknesses of previous studies and consider the implications for their findings. Keep in mind that your review should include a critical evaluation of the literature on your topic and an assessment of the soundness of the findings reported. (See Chapter 6.)

ORGANIZATION OF THE MAIN BODY OF THE CHAPTER

The content of the review demonstrates your grasp and understanding of the current state of knowledge in your field of study. However, that knowledge should not be an "information dump," where individual studies, theories, ideas, and concepts are piled together in a muddled display. Rather, you should present a holistic narrative where the literature sources are woven together in a sound organization to reveal logical relationships and connections.

There are several methods of structuring the themes in the main body of the literature; six of the most commonly used methods are: (1) dividing the content around distinct themes; (2) developing the structure chronologically; (3) separating the theoretical contemplation from the empirical discussion; (4) surveying the theoretical literature first, then presenting a methodological discussion; (5) using a systematic review organization; and (6) applying a hermeneutic–phenomenological structure. Regardless of your choice of organizational structure, consider the writing of the main body of the literature as a "funnel." The discussion in this funnel starts out broad, examining the topic from a wide angle; eventually the narrative is narrowed down and is focused on those themes and subthemes that are most relevant to your problem statement and research questions. (See Chapter 7 for our expanded discussion on organizing the review.)

PRESENTING A PERSUASIVE ARGUMENT IN THE MAIN BODY OF THE CHAPTER

Your writing in the literature review puts forward a particular argument that is developed throughout the narrative. This argument is comprised of a series of propositions that are convincingly supported by empirical research and/or theoretical sources. Each section of your literature review should advance or provide a context for your review's central argument; each paragraph should be related to the major claims that are building the section's arguments; and the sentences in each paragraph should highlight the points that make up the propositions presented in the paragraph. Combined together logically and clearly, all these claims and propositions make up a coherent case designed to persuade your readers that the argument you proposed is justified and convincing. (See Chapter 8 for our expanded discussion on developing arguments and supporting claims.)

Summary and Discussion

The summary and discussion section is the bridge that links the knowledge you have gained through the review of the literature and the research you plan to conduct. You construct this bridge by summarizing what you have learned through your review, evaluating current knowledge on the topic, and proposing a rationale for your own study.

SYNTHESIZING AND INTERPRETING THE SOURCES IN THE MAIN BODY OF THE CHAPTER

When organizing the review, you do not want to merely summarize and report the sources you have chosen. Rather, you should synthesize and interpret the sources by revealing the meaning you have made from the texts. In the synthesis and interpretation process, you weave together sources, find connections among them, and look for patterns and trends. Additionally, despite the fact the review is based on what other authors and researchers have written, in the synthesis and interpretation process you want to expand current knowledge by advancing new perspectives, discovering new models, providing unique ideas and concepts, expanding existing explanations, or even offering an original theory.

You accomplish this synthesis and interpretation process by grouping together and by comparing and contrasting theories, concepts, methodologies, and findings in order to identify how they relate to or differ from each other. You recognize and address conflicting positions, contradicting evidence, inconsistencies, or rival explanations, and offer possible reasons for these. You also demonstrate a critical stance by assessing theories and particular perspectives, and evaluating specific studies or groups of studies. (See Chapter 9 for our expanded discussion on the interpretation and synthesis of sources.)

SUMMARIZING WHAT YOU HAVE LEARNED THROUGH THE REVIEW

In this section, you look back at your literature review and remind the reader what you aimed to achieve in this chapter. You briefly summarize the major ideas, concepts, and claims; highlight patterns; and point out key findings and their meaning.

EVALUATING CURRENT KNOWLEDGE ON THE TOPIC

Here you highlight the main points of criticism of previous work conducted on our topic that you have discussed in the main body of the literature review. You acknowledge deficiencies and shortcomings; point out tensions and inconsistencies; and identify gaps, limitations, and unresolved problems that provide a justification for your own investigation.

PROPOSING A RATIONALE FOR YOUR OWN STUDY

This section leads the reader logically and coherently to the objectives of your study. You provide an explanation of how your research may contribute to the field and extend current knowledge by filling a gap in the existing body of knowledge, overcoming current limitations, or resolving existing conflicts.

Table 12.2 (p. 257) presents a summary of the components that you may include in the literature review chapter.

TABLE 12.2. An Outline of the Major Components in Chapter 2 (the Literature Review)	
Introduction to the literature review chapter	▪ A brief statement of what you intend to achieve in your review ▪ Review organization: major themes ▪ Type of literature review you have chosen to write (systematic, traditional–narrative, hermeneutic–phenomenological) (this component is optional) ▪ Inclusion/exclusion criteria ▪ Literature search: keywords, databases, and other parameters (mostly for systematic reviews)
Main body of the literature review	▪ Content: historical framework, theoretical framework, methodological and research findings ▪ Effective organization ▪ Synthesis of the sources ▪ Persuasive proposed argument
Summary and discussion	▪ Summary of the main points learned through the review ▪ Evaluating current knowledge on the topic ▪ Proposing a rationale for your own study

||||||||||||||||||||||||||||||||||THE LITERATURE REVIEW WITHIN THE THESIS OR DISSERTATION

Writing the literature review is not a task that is completed once you finish writing Chapter 2. Rather, it is important that you revisit and continually remain fully engaged with the scholarly work of others throughout the process of writing the thesis, dissertation, or grant proposal. The theories, ideas, methodologies, and findings that you discuss in the literature review chapter extend to the other chapters and have an integral and practical role in constructing them (Boote & Beile, 2005; Glense, 2018; Hart, 1998; Marshall & Rossman, 2011; Ravitch & Riggan, 2017).

The literature review offers a frame of reference for planning and executing your own study. Methodological decisions regarding your research design and the selection of particular data collection methods should logically and conceptually flow from your review. The review may also inform you about how to analyze your own data by providing the constructs and categories for organizing and filtering the data, helping you choose what you want to emphasize, and assisting you in explaining and interpreting your study's findings. Your discussion in the literature review is used to validate your study's findings by comparing and contrasting them with what is currently known, and showing how your research is rooted in. and contributes to, the body of scholarship in your field of study.

The influential role of the literature review is evident in a dissertation written by Gina, a doctoral student of education. In her review, which was centered on three approaches to democratic citizenship education, she compared the theory underlying each approach, discussed the pedagogical implications and practices that distinguish each, and critically described the assessment of these approaches as reported by other researchers. Gina's literature review served as a context for her own case study, in which she investigated how the values of democratic citizenship are integrated explicitly and implicitly in the curriculum and daily life of three middle schools in a Midwestern suburb. Her research design and data collection strategies, and her analysis and interpretation, were linked to the literature on these theories. In Gina's reflections on the meaning of her research findings, she compared and contrasted how the ideas, curriculum, and assessment of those three approaches were reflected in what actually took place in the daily life of each of the three educational settings.

At times, when you discuss your findings and conclusions, you may realize that your research yields unexpected results. Similarly, you may, while conducting the study, encounter unanticipated complexities that cause you to view your topic in a new light. In such cases, Ravitch and Riggan (2017) suggest that you revisit your literature review and consider shifting the focus somewhat, or even introduce new elements to your previous narrative. Doing so, Ravitch and Riggan assert, leads to a discovery of new insights and valuable contributions to the ongoing scholarly conversation.

Similarly, Ridley (2012) proposes that researchers continue reading relevant sources until the final completion of their dissertation work. Following Ridley, we suggest that you keep watching for new publications on your topic, be open to new ideas and new findings, and—whenever appropriate—integrate current scholarship on your topic into your work.

An example of a need to revisit one's literature review is the dissertation of Paul Reiff (2016) whose work was mentioned before. Reiff wrote a phenomenological study on high school students' experience of beauty. Drawing from classical and contemporary poets, philosophers, and curriculum theorists, Paul presented in his literature review a rich and extensive historical and philosophical overview of the concepts of *beauty, aesthetics*, and the *experience of wonder*. However, at the data interpretation stage, Paul encountered an unexpected disconnect between the ideas he discussed in his literature review and his students' understanding of the role of beauty in their lives. When his students talked about beauty, they focused on relationships and friendships, on overcoming adversities, and on discovery of self. Paul was confounded by this disconnect between his understanding of beauty and that of his students. At the same time, he found inspiration and joy in grappling with these different world views. He revisited his literature review and added a section that reconsidered the idea of beauty through the concept of "awakening" (Greene, 1978), which refers to the use of imagination and arts in waking one's mind, spirit, and self-awareness. In his interpretation of his findings, Reiff discussed the meaning of his research results through the lens of the unexpected revelation and insights and through the concept of awakening as experienced by his students.

The Literature Review in Different Formats of Dissertations and Theses

The knowledge, understandings, and insights gained through the review of the literature sources are integrated and interwoven throughout the thesis, dissertation, or grant work. The typical literature review appears as a single and distinctive chapter, which is then followed by three chapters (on method, results, and discussion). This structural format is most commonly used by doctoral and master's level students. However, this is not the only possible format. In the following section, we highlight additional formats you may consider for writing your literature review.

Platridge (2002) identifies four basic formats of including the literature review in dissertations and theses in the social sciences and humanities: traditional simple, traditional complex, topic-based, and compilation of articles. In each of these patterns, the literature review is structured differently in relation to the rest of the chapters.

Traditional Simple Format

This format, as mentioned above, comprises five chapters. The second chapter is a separate literature review which is followed by three chapters, all dedicated to a single study. This type of dissertation follows the generic structure referred to as ILMRC (Introduction, Literature Review, Methods, Results, Discussion). Dissertations or theses typically used in the fields of science and medicine also belong to the simple traditional pattern, although the literature review in such dissertations appears as part of the introduction (LMRC format).

Traditional Complex Format

This format is an expanded version of the traditional simple dissertation pattern (Thompson, 1999). What distinguishes the traditional complex from the traditional simple pattern is that it contains several related, though independent, studies. Each of these studies is presented in the IMRC (introduction, methods, results, conclusion) structure. These individual studies are connected by a single literature review that serves as an overarching umbrella. This dissertation pattern is often used in scientific fields and the behavioral sciences.

An example is a study by Rachel, a student in psychology, on the topic of the development of self-concept in school-age children. After reviewing the literature on this topic, Rachel posts three research questions, and each of these questions is the focus of a separate study that she has conducted. In the first study, she administered a self-report rating scale to 200 children in urban areas in the Southwest. In the second study, Rachel compared the self-concept of children in three different cultural communities using a survey completed by their parents. In the third study, Rachel assessed the impact of social media sites, such as Facebook and Twitter, on children's self-image, using a self-rating survey. Each of these studies is reported on in a separate chapter that includes an introduction, methods, results, and discussion. The last chapter presents a general discussion that ties together the findings of the individual studies and provides suggestions for psychologists and other practitioners who work with children.

Topic-Based Format

This structural pattern of dissertations uses themes or topics to structure the chapters. A dissertation that follows this pattern does not contain a separate and independent chapter for the literature review but rather the content of the literature review is interspersed throughout the chapters. Distinct chapters for methods and results are usually not included in this format. Typically, the dissertation or thesis begins with an introduction chapter, followed by topic-based chapters, and ends with a general discussion and conclusion chapter. The topic-based pattern is mostly used in nonempirical research, such as theoretical, theological, and philosophical studies (Carter, Kelly, & Brailsford, 2012).

An example of the topic-based pattern can be seen in the dissertation written by Jason Francel (2015) titled *The War on Education: A Prisoner's Dilemma*. Box 12.5 provides a brief description of each chapter of his dissertation.

BOX 12.5. A Topic-Based Pattern

Chapter 1: The Disabled Knower. Francel introduces the dissertation topic through an auto-ethnography that immerses the reader in his experience as a teacher and a doctoral student.

Chapter 2: A Hermeneutic Discourse from the Aesthetics of Democracy. In this chapter, hermeneutic and aesthetics discourse is used to propose a more horizontal form of knowledge.

Chapter 3: Essentially Democratic: The Death of Progressivism in Education. Through the readings of progressive and essentialist writers, Francel examines whether there has been a truly democratic progress in education.

Chapter 4: The Prison. In this chapter, Francel describes the classroom as the walls that imprison the learners from logically constructed progressions of language.

Chapter 5: Out of Sight Out of Mind. The writer considers how our educational language imprisons the learner, who becomes captive to a system that falsely casts images of progress.

Source: Francel (2015).

Compilation of Articles

This format, also known as *thesis for publication,* is composed of a series of chapters; each comprises a different study, essay, or article written by the doctoral candidate. Each chapter is independent of the rest and includes its own review of literature (Dong, 1998). These chapters were already published as journal articles, conference papers, or book chapters, or are being considered for publication. To enhance the cohesiveness of this type of dissertation, it is recommended that an introduction and a conclusion chapter be included. The introduction provides a wide contextual background of the current state of knowledge. The conclusion chapter demonstrates a comprehensive summary of the chapters and may include a synthesis of their conclusions and implications for the field.

What distinguishes this type of dissertation is that there is an expectation that its writers are "experts writing for experts" (Platridge, 2002, p. 132). The focus of these writers is not on demonstrating their knowledge to their dissertation committee but rather on their contributions to the current body of scholarly knowledge in their field (Boote & Beile, 2005).

Box 12.6 presents Magrini's (2014) rationale for choosing a compilation of articles pattern for his dissertation.

BOX 12.6. An Excerpt from a Rationale for Choosing a Compilation of Articles Pattern for a Dissertation

I have chosen a non-traditional format for my dissertation termed "thesis by publication," or "compilation dissertation," for several reasons, not the least of which is that it will allow me to utilize the published research. . . . A *thesis by publication* will "make it possible to disseminate the work to a larger audience," and also prepare me for the type of communication I "will be expected to do throughout [my] career" (Duke & Beck, 1999, p. 31). And, typically, as Boote and Beile (2005) point out, dissertations in the compilation format "contain much less writing that seems to serve the purpose of merely displaying the author's knowledge" and are rather concerned with making viable and substantial contributions to the existing body of scholarly literature in the field (p. 10). . . . As a "thesis by publication," outside of Chapter 1, which presents for the reader a holistic view of the methodological, philosophical, historical, and linguistic context from out of which the research emerges and returns, the rest of the chapters are individual published essays-articles that are works of "stand-alone" scholarship. However, in keeping with the formal-thematic structure of this type of dissertation, it is necessary to center the article-chapters around, by relating them to, the overarching theme I have introduced, that of the *human being as original learner,* this in order to bring these chapters together to form a cohesive manuscript.

Source: Magrini (2014).

TABLE 12.3. A Summary of the Literature Review Patterns within Different Dissertation and Thesis Formats	
Pattern	**Description of format**
Traditional simple pattern	Contains five chapters, referred to as ILMRC. The literature review is a separate chapter, followed by three chapters that are dedicated to a single study.
Traditional complex pattern	Includes a single literature review that serves as an overarching umbrella to several related, though independent, studies. Each of these studies is presented in the IMRC structure.
Topic-based pattern	Begins with an introduction chapter and ends with a general discussion chapter. Does not contain a separate literature review chapter; rather, the review of the literature is interspersed throughout the chapters.
Compilation of articles	Composed of a series of independent chapters, each comprising a different study published or presented in a conference by the dissertation writer. All chapters include their own literature reviews.

Table 12.3 summarizes the patterns of literature review in different formats of dissertations and theses.

WRITING TIPS AND RHETORICAL DEVICES

The coherence of your writing is one of the most important factors that contributes to the quality of your literature review and to the understanding of your argument. This means that your narrative is held together effectively, the different sections and paragraphs are clearly connected, and the ideas flow smoothly, logically, and purposefully.

As a writer, it is your responsibility to make the literature review as crisply clear as possible for the readers. Following are some writing tips and rhetorical devices that may enhance your readers' ability to move effortlessly through your text and navigate with greater ease the long and complex narrative of the literature review chapter.

One Idea per Paragraph

Every paragraph should have only one main idea; therefore, when you introduce a new idea, you should start a new paragraph. This main idea is introduced in a key sentence that addresses the paragraph's main point. The other sentences in the paragraph may support, clarify, illustrate, and provide details that reinforce this key sentence.

> **BOX 12.7.** A Paragraph That Includes a Major Idea and Lists Parts of That Idea
>
> When choosing the style for your literature review, be cognizant of several factors. These include: (1) your academic field's norms; (2) the audience you are writing for; (3) the type of literature review you are writing; and (4) your own orientation as a writer.

The main idea in the paragraph in Box 12.7 may include several points related to that idea. For example, in the following paragraph the writer offers advice on how to choose the style of the literature review. The writer presents the major idea in the first sentence and then lists the factors that are parts of that idea. However, because long paragraphs are hard to follow, if these individual factors are later explained and discussed at length, you should create a new paragraph for each.

While the key sentence in which the main idea is introduced may be presented anywhere in the paragraph, it is often recommended that you put it at the beginning of the paragraph. Starting the paragraph with the key sentence ensures that the readers know what the main idea of the paragraph is. Paragraphs should not be too long or too short; each paragraph should contain at least two sentences, unless the single sentence introduces the text that follows, such as a list, table, or figure.

When reviewing your paragraphs, make sure that there are no paragraphs that repeat and duplicate the same ideas. There is nothing more tedious than reading the same claim, concept, or idea over and over again with minimal variation. If a similar claim, concept, or idea runs through more than one paragraph (whether in consecutive paragraphs, in paragraphs in proximity to each other, or in different sections of the review), read and compare them closely. Check whether any of those paragraphs include specific nuances, present other information, or provide additional supporting evidence, rather than simply repeat each other. If, however, you recognize that these paragraphs, although they may be worded differently, propose exactly the same claim, concept, or idea, consider combining them into one. This will allow you to pick and choose the best-worded phrases or sentences from those paragraphs, keep the elements that best reflect or support your idea, and eliminate the rest.

Transitional Markers

Literature reviews for theses, dissertations, and grant proposals tend to be lengthy and complex. It may be challenging for the readers to see the logical linkage between the different themes and sections and to realize how they all connect to each other and build a cohesive argument.

To enhance your readers' ability to see the cohesiveness of your writing, use transitional words or expressions. Transitional markers (1) link together sentences, paragraphs, and sections in your review; (2) indicate the connections you are making; and (3) mark the progression of your ideas. The transitional devices may point out that you are making an additional point (e.g., *moreover, furthermore, additionally*), comparing and contrasting (e.g., *on the other hand, similarly, by comparison*), sequencing (e.g., *first, second, third*), or showing cause and effect (e.g., *as a result, consequently, because*).

The transitional devices can be a single word (e.g., *next, therefore*), short phrase (e.g., *as noted earlier, it is often argued*), or full sentence (e.g., *"The issues raised by the researchers have shed light on the complexity of the idea of. . . . This point is frequently overlooked, usually in favor of the more familiar concept of. . . ."*).

Such transitional words or phrases serve as textual cues for your readers that help them understand the logical relationships among your sentences or paragraphs and provide them with guidelines on how to piece together your ideas. They can be seen as bridges that enhance the readers' ability to sense the flow of your ideas and their logical organization.

Repeated Words and Phrases

Repeating some words and phrases from a prior paragraph is another way of ensuring that one paragraph flows smoothly into the next. This device links the paragraphs and indicates which particular point you are continuing to develop or expand.

Box 12.8 illustrates how this type of repetition can provide a transition from one paragraph to the next. The repeated words are italicized in this example.

On the other hand, avoid repeating the same word again and again within a paragraph. Instead, alternative synonymous words may be used. For example, to avoid repeating the word "often," you may use "usually," or "frequently."

BOX 12.8. A Repetition of Words and a Phrase to Provide a Transition from One Paragraph to the Next

Taylor and Kilgus (2014) discussed the importance of social–emotional learning for students' academic performance. They highlight programs that develop social–emotional skills through a positive support system. *Growth mindset* is one such *program* that can be *used* in the *classroom*.

The *growth mindset program* is currently being *used* and taught in many *classrooms*. It was developed by Dweck (2016) and refers to the way people think about themselves, their learning, motivation, and success. . . .

Navigating Devices

As you are trying to help your readers follow your literature review narrative, consider yourself a tour guide that assists them in navigating their way through the complexity of your writing. Two tools you may use to navigate your reader through your narrative are: (1) signposts and (2) summaries of major sections or themes.

Signposts

The signposts serve as transitions from one section to the next and, as the name suggests, signal logical movement in the narrative. You begin each major section with a sentence or two that points out to the reader what will be unfolding in the coming discussion and what to anticipate. The signpost often explains how the issue at the center of the upcoming section logically follows and builds upon what was previously discussed. An example of a signpost can be seen in Box 12.9.

Summary of Major Sections or Themes

End each discussion of a major section or a theme with a summary that reiterates in a concise way the major points argued and creates a logical segue to the section that follows. These summaries that are interspersed throughout the literature review allow readers to understand how the sections are ordered and how the different parts build the literature review's arguments. Box 12.10 shows an example of a summary of a central section.

BOX 12.9. A Signpost

In the previous section I discussed the theory that underlies. . . . I am now turning your attention to the implications of this theoretical perspective for practice. The upcoming section begins with. . . . It then goes on to deliberate . . . and finally it will. . . .

BOX 12.10. A Summary of a Central Section

In summary, understanding the concept of culture, as discussed in this section, provides a theoretical basis for examining. . . . The deliberative stance implied by this approach yields a vision of authentic discourse, in which plurality is nurtured and empowered. With this understanding, I am turning now to the next section where I explore the . . . of urban youth community.

Headings and Subheadings

The use of headings and subheadings provides another tool that contributes to the cohesiveness and flow of your literature review. Headings and subheadings separate and identify the sections in your review, reveal the structure of the narrative, identify the main issues in each section, and help to advance the various strands of your argument. The headings and subheadings convey the hierarchy of the themes and subthemes of your work, allowing the reader to follow your writing more easily.

Construct the headings and subheading from the key terms or words that highlight and distinguish the essence of each section and subsection of your narrative. Format the headings and subheadings according to the writing style you follow (e.g., APA, MLA, and Chicago Style). Adhere to the rules consistently throughout the literature review (as well as the other chapters of your work).

The sixth edition of the APA publication manual, for example, offers guidelines for five heading labels, although literature review writers usually use only two, three, or four levels. Regardless of the number of levels, always use the headings in order, beginning with level 1 without skipping any level. Table 12.4 describes the different heading and subheading levels according to APA style (*https://owl.english.purdue.edu/owl/resource/560/16/*) and Box 12.11 (p. 267) presents a diagram of APA headings and subheadings.

Summary Tables

Finally, some writers find it beneficial to summarize information in the literature review by using tables. They assert that tables are an effective way to summarize and display information from a variety of sources. While tables are particularly effective for displaying statistical results, they also can be appropriate for comparing two or more theoretical perspectives or summarizing results of qualitative studies such as listing themes and patterns in each research study.

Keep in mind that these summary tables cannot speak for themselves but rather serve as a tool to illustrate and support what is described in depth in the

TABLE 12.4. Different Headings and Subheading Levels According to APA Style

Level of heading	Format
1	Centered, boldface, uppercase and lowercase heading.
2	Left-aligned, boldface, uppercase and lowercase heading.
3	Indented, boldface, lowercase heading with a period. Begin text after the period.
4	Indented, boldface, italicized, lowercase heading with a period. Begin text after the period.
5	Indented, italicized, lowercase heading with a period. Begin text after the period.

> **BOX 12.11.** A Diagram of APA Headings and Subheadings
>
>
>
> **Level One Heading**
>
>
>
> Text begins here . . .
>
> **Level Two Heading**
>
> Text begins here . . .
>
> > **Level three.** Text begins here . . .
> >
> > ***Level four.*** Text begins here . . .
> >
> > *Level five.* Text begins here . . .

text. In your narrative, you need to introduce the table by pointing out to the reader what to pay attention to and how the information in the table is relevant to your proposed argument. Additionally, don't forget to label and identify each table.

Table 12.5 summarizes the writing tips and rhetorical devices that are used to enhance the cohesiveness of the literature review narrative.

TABLE 12.5. A Summary of Writing Tips and Rhetorical Devices Used to Strengthen the Cohesiveness of Literature Review Writing

Tip	Description
One idea per paragraph	Every paragraph should have only one main idea that addresses the paragraph's major point.
Transitional markers	Transitional markers link together sentences, paragraphs, and sections in the review.
Repeated phrases	Repeating phrases from a prior paragraph links paragraphs and indicates which particular point is further developed or expanded.
Signposts	The signposts at the beginning of new sections signal logical movement in the narrative and point out what will be discussed next.
Summary of major sections or themes	Major sections or themes end with summaries that reiterate the narrative's main points and offer segues to the section that follows.
Headings and subheadings	Headings and subheadings reveal the structure of the narrative, identify the main themes and subthemes, and convey their hierarchy.
Summary tables	Summary tables concisely display information from a variety of sources, compare the results of different studies, and juxtapose theoretical perspectives.

LITERATURE REVIEW ASSESSMENT MATRICES ||||||||||||||||||||||||||||||||||||||||||||||||||||||||||||

Congratulations! After working hard for weeks, months, and perhaps even years, you have finished writing your literature review from beginning to end! As we mentioned before (see Chapter 10), writing the literature review is a process that involves revisiting and rewriting your work over and over again. Now, you are ready to reread your review and do a final editing of the complete manuscript.

We end the chapter and this book with six assessment matrices (Tables 12.6– 12.11, pp. 269–274) that are designed to assist you in undertaking the final editing. You can accomplish this task by yourself, with your writing group, or with a friend or colleague.

We suggest that before you start the final editing process, you familiarize yourself with these assessment matrices. As you can see, the categories in the matrices relate to the entire literature review rather than to specific chapters or sections. These categories are (A) introduction, (B) topic knowledge and understanding, (C) organization and final discussion, (D) arguments, synthesis, and coherency, (E) writer voice and rhetorical devices, and (F) formatting and writing mechanics.

Next, read your review, from beginning to end, and take notes on the different elements in the matrices. Reviewing and revising your work is a dynamic process that evolves through different iterations. Therefore, you will probably need to reevaluate previous comments you made, add comments on certain points in the tables, or revise your earlier notes. Your notes and comments will assist you in the ongoing process of improving your work, refining the organization of your writing, polishing your style, and optimizing the clarity of your text.

Part A—Introduction

Part A of the assessment matrix focuses on the introduction section of your literature review. Chapter 3 and a section of this chapter include an in-depth discussion of elements of this category.

TABLE 12.6. Literature Review Assessment Matrix: Part A—Introduction	
Assessment criteria	**Comments**
1. The opening grabs the reader's attention.	
2. The problem statement is clear and concise and unambiguously articulates the focus of the study.	
3. The purpose statement presents clearly and succinctly the objectives of the study.	
4. The research question is specific, focused, clear, and answerable.	
5. The terms are well defined and consistently used throughout the text.	
6. The significance of the topic and its contributions to the field and/or society are clearly articulated.	
7. The topic is contextualized within the contemporary, theoretical, and/or historical issues surrounding it.	
8. Possible biases and subjectivity toward the topic are discussed.	
9. The scope of the study and its boundaries are discussed.	
10. An overview of the chapters that follow is presented.	

Part B—Topic Knowledge and Understanding

Part B of the assessment matrix focuses on the topic knowledge category of your literature review. The assessment criteria are based on in-depth discussion of elements of this category in Chapter 5 and a section of this chapter.

TABLE 12.7. Literature Review Assessment Matrix: Part B—Topic Knowledge and Understanding	
Assessment criteria	Comments
1. The criteria for inclusion and exclusion of sources are clearly articulated.	
2. The sources are relevant and contribute to the reader's understanding of the research topic.	
3. Appropriate primary and secondary sources are used.	
4. The topic is placed within the historical context of the research area.	
5. The topic is situated within contemporary contexts and demonstrates knowledge of current publications.	
6. Theoretical perspectives are presented, explained, and compared.	
7. Methodological assumptions and research techniques employed in previous studies are described and critiqued.	
8. Main scholars, authoritative writers, and seminal studies in the field are cited.	
9. Multiple perspectives on the topic are presented, discussed, and evaluated.	
10. Debates, controversies, and agreements among researchers are discussed, and conflicting positions are presented.	

Part C—Organization and Final Discussion

The focus of Part C of the assessment matrix is on the organization and final section of the literature review. The criteria in this category are based on in-depth discussions in Chapter 7 and the last part of Chapter 8, as well as a section in this chapter.

TABLE 12.8. Literature Review Assessment Matrix: Part C—Organization and Final Discussion	
Assessment criteria	**Comments**
1. A logical organization of the review is evident.	
2. The content is divided around distinct themes and subthemes.	
3. The flow from one idea to another is smooth, logical, and effective.	
4. The review is organized from a broad discussion to a narrower and more focused examination.	
5. The literature review leads logically to the writer's own research.	
6. The literature review ends with a brief summary showing what was learned through the review.	
7. Ideas that were not discussed in the literature review are not included in the summary of the literature review.	
8. Current knowledge on the topic is evaluated in the final section of the literature review and discrepancies, inconsistencies, and gaps are pointed out.	
9. A rationale for the writer's own study is proposed in the summary of the literature review.	
10. Suggestions to overcome past problems are offered in the final section.	

Part D—Arguments, Synthesis, and Coherency

The focus of Part D of the assessment matrix is on building an argument, synthesis of the sources, coherency of the writing, and critical reading of the studies. The criteria in this category are based on in-depth discussions in Chapters 6, 8, and 9, as well as a section in this chapter.

TABLE 12.9. Literature Review Assessment Matrix: Part D—Arguments, Synthesis, Coherency, and Critical Reading	
Assessment criteria	**Comments**
1. The claims are logically built step by step to formulate the main argument.	
2. The argument and claims are well developed and are supported by evidence.	
3. The major argument is developed in a way that is coherent and relevant to the research question.	
4. The argument presents persuasively and logically the standpoint of the writer on the topic.	
5. Existing literature is effectively synthesized to advance, expand, or offer a new perspective on the topic.	
6. The synthesis compares and contrasts ideas, theories, and findings to highlight patterns, explanations, or conclusions.	
7. The synthesis is carried out with a critical stance that questions theories and ideas.	
8. The synthesis demonstrates coherency of ideas and the writer's perspective and subjectivity.	
9. The review reflects a critical evaluation of the sources and an assessment of the findings.	
10. The reviewer shows respect toward researchers whose studies are criticized.	

Part E—Writer Voice and Rhetorical Devices

Part E of the assessment matrix centers on writer voice and rhetoric. The criteria in this category are based on in-depth discussions in Chapter 10 and sections of this chapter.

TABLE 12.10. Literature Review Assessment Matrix: Part E—Writer Voice and Rhetorical Devices	
Assessment criteria	**Comments**
1. The writer's voice is authoritative and present.	
2. The writer's ideas are differentiated from those of the reviewed authors.	
3. Each paragraph contains a complete and logical thought.	
4. Transitions link together sentences, paragraphs, and sections in the review.	
5. The signposts at the beginnings of new sections signal logical movements in the narrative and point out what will be discussed next.	
6. Central sections or themes end with summaries that reiterate the narrative's major points and offer effective transition to the section that follows.	
7. When appropriate, graphics, figures, and tables are used to illustrate and summarize points.	
8. Levels of headings clearly indicate the text organization and relationships among the different parts of the review.	
9. Alternative synonymous words are used to avoid repeating the same words over and over in the same paragraph.	

Part F—Formulating and Writing Mechanics

Part F of the assessment matrix focuses on formatting the text and on writing mechanics. The criteria in this category are based on in-depth discussion in Chapter 11, as well as suggestions for formatting and writing mechanics throughout the book.

TABLE 12.11. Literature Review Assessment Matrix: Part F—Formatting and Writing Mechanics	
Assessment criteria	**Comments**
1. The margins and font size are set correctly, and page headers/numbers are inserted.	
2. The text is written according to a chosen writing style manual.	
3. In-text references and citations match the reference list or bibliography at the end of the review.	
4. Sentences present coherent thoughts and are not too long.	
5. Correct syntax, spelling, and punctuation are used throughout the text.	
6. Terms used for the first time are spelled out, whereas acronyms may be used subsequently.	
7. Consistent verb tenses are used and there is agreement of verbs and subject, and verbs nouns.	
8. Italics, quotation marks, capitalization, hyphenation, and abbreviations are appropriately used.	
9. Quotes, tables, and statistical findings are introduced and explained in the text.	
10. All the electronic links in the text and references are active and accurate.	

CHAPTER SUMMARY

1. The review of the literature has a major role in the first two chapters of a thesis or dissertation: Chapter 1 (Introduction) and Chapter 2 (Literature Review).

2. The introduction chapter (Chapter 1) should provoke your reader's interest, state clearly the topic and purpose of your study, define its major terms and concepts, explain its significance, describe its contexts, present the research questions, delineate its scope, and outline a road map.

3. There is no single way of formatting the literature review, but generally it is divided into an *introduction, main body,* and *summary and discussion.*

4. The introduction describes what you achieve in your literature review and may include the criteria for inclusion and exclusion of sources.

5. In writing the main body of the review the focus should be on four aspects: (a) content of the review, (b) effective organization, (c) coherent synthesis and interpretation of sources, and (d) persuasive proposed argument.

6. The summary and discussion sections form the bridge to the research you plan to conduct. It includes a summary of what was learned in the review, evaluation of current knowledge, and a rationale for your own study.

7. Writing the literature review is not a task that is completed once you finish writing it; rather, you should revisit and remain engaged in the work of others throughout your scholarly writing process.

8. There are four basic formats of including the literature review in dissertations and theses in the social sciences and humanities: traditional simple, traditional complex, topic based, and compilation of articles. In each of those formats the review is structured differently.

9. As a writer, it is your responsibility to make the literature review as crisply clear as possible for the readers. Writing tips and rhetorical devices include one idea per paragraph, transitional markers, repeating phrases, navigating devices, headings and subheadings, and summary tables.

10. Revise and refine your writing using these six assessment matrices that focus on the following categories: (a) introduction, (b) topic knowledge and understanding, (c) organization and final discussion, (d) argument construction and synthesis, (e) writer voice and coherency, and (f) formatting and writing mechanics.

References

American Psychological Association. (2010). *Publication manual of the American Psychological Association* (6th ed.). Washington, DC: Author.

Atkins, S., Lewin, S., Smith, H., Engel, M., Fretheim, A., & Volmink, J. (2008). Conducting a meta-ethnography of qualitative literature: Lessons learnt. *BMC Medical Research Methodology, 8*(21), 1–10.

Axelrod, R. B., & Cooper, C. R. (2012). *Axelrod and Cooper concise guide to writing* (6th ed.). Boston: Belford/St. Martin.

Bakhtin, M. M. (1981). *The dialogic imagination: Four essays* (M. Holquist, Ed., C. Emerson & M. Holquist, Trans.). Austin: University of Texas Press.

Bandura, A. (1977). *Social learning theory.* Englewood Cliffs, NJ: Prentice Hall.

Barnett-Page, E., & Thomas, J. (2009). Methods for the synthesis of qualitative research: A critical review. *BMC Medical Research Methodology, 9,* 59.

Barrett, F. J., Powley, E. H., & Pearce, B. (2011). Hermeneutic philosophy and organizational theory. In H. Tsoukas & R. Chia (Eds.), *Philosophy and organization theory: Vol. 32. Research in the sociology of organizations* (pp. 181–213). Bingley, UK: Emerald.

Battany-Saltikov, J. (2012). *How to do a systematic literature review in nursing: A step-by-step guide.* Berkshire, UK: Open University Press.

Bazeley, P. (2013). *Qualitative data analysis: Practical strategies.* Thousand Oaks, CA: SAGE.

Berg, B. L., & Lune, H. (2011). *Qualitative research methods for the social sciences* (8th ed.). Essex, UK: Pearson.

Black, T. R. (1999). *Doing quantitative research in the social sciences: An integrated approach to research design, measurement and statistics.* Thousand Oaks, CA: SAGE.

Blumberg, B., Cooper, D. R., & Schindler, P. S. (2008). *Business research method* (2nd ed.). Berkshire, UK: McGraw-Hill.

Boell, S. K., & Cecez-Kecmanovic, D. (2010). Literature reviews and the hermeneutic circle. *Australian Academic and Research Libraries, 41*(2), 129–144.

Boell, S. K., & Cecez-Kecmanovic, D. (2014). A hermeneutic approach for conducting literature review and literature search. *Communications of the Association for Information Systems, 34,* 257–286.

Bogdan, R. C., & Biklen, S. K. (2006). *Qualitative research in education: An introduction to theory and methods* (5th ed.). Needham Heights, MA: Allyn & Bacon.

Boote, D. N., & Beile, P. (2005). Scholars before researchers: On the centrality of literature review in dissertation preparation. *Educational Researchers, 34*(6), 3–15.

Booth, A., Sutton, A., & Papaioannou, D. (2016). *Systematic approaches to a successful literature review* (2nd ed.). Thousand Oaks, CA: SAGE.

Booth, W. C., Colomb G. G., & Williams, J. M. (2008). *The craft of research* (3rd ed.). Chicago: University of Chicago Press.

Brannen, J. (2005). Mixed methods: The entry of qualitative and quantitative approaches into the research process. *International Journal of Social Research Methodology, 8*(3), 173–184.

Britten, N., Campbell, R., Pope, C., Donovan, J., Morgan, M., & Pill, R. (2002). Using meta ethnography to synthesize qualitative research: A worked example. *Journal of Health Services Research and Policy, 7*(4), 209–215.

Bronfenbrenner, U. (1979). *The ecology of human development: Experiments by nature and design.* Cambridge, MA: Harvard University Press.

Bruce, C. S. (2001). Interpreting the scope of their literature reviews: Significance differences in research students' concerns. *New Library World, 102*(4), 158–166.

Campbell, R., Pound, P., Morgan, M., Daker-White, G., Britten, N., Pill, R., et al. (2011). Evaluating meta-ethnography: Systematic analysis and synthesis of qualitative research. *Health Technology Assessment, 15*(43), 1–64.

Campbell, R., Pound, P., Pope, C., Britten, N., Pill, R., Morgan, M., et al. (2003). Evaluating meta-ethnography: A synthesis of qualitative research on lay experiences of diabetes and diabetes care. *Social Science and Medicine, 56*(4), 671–684.

Card, N. A. (2015). *Applied meta-analysis for social science research.* New York: Guilford Press.

Carnwell R., & Daly, W. (2001) Strategies for the construction of a critical review of the literature. *Nurse Education Practice, 1*(2), 57–63.

Carter, S., Kelly, F., & Brailsford, I. (2012). *Structuring your research thesis.* London: Palgrave Macmillan.

Cazden, C. B. (1993). Vygotski, Hymes and Bakhtin: From words to utterance and voice. In E. M. Minick & E. Forman (Eds.), *Contexts for learning: Sociocultural dynamic of children's development* (pp. 197–212). New York: Oxford University Press.

Chicago Manual of Style (17th ed.). (2017). Chicago: University of Chicago Press. Retrieved from *www.chicagomanualofstyle.org/home.html.*

Coburn, C. E., & Penuel, W. R. (2016). Research–practice partnerships in education: Outcomes, dynamics, and open questions. *Educational Researcher, 45*(1), 48–54.

Coffin, C., Curry, M. J., Goodman, S., Hewings, A., Lillis, T. M., & Swann, J. (2003). *Teaching academic writing: A toolkit for higher education.* New York: Routledge.

Cooper, H. (1984). *The integrative research review: A systematic approach.* Beverley Hills, CA: SAGE.

Cooper, H. (1988). Organizing knowledge synthesis: A taxonomy of literature reviews. *Knowledge in Society, 1*(1), 104–128.

Cooper, H. (1998). *Synthesizing research: A guide for literature reviews* (3rd ed.). Thousand Oaks, CA: SAGE.

Cooper, H. (2010). *Research synthesis and meta-analysis: A step-by-step approach* (3rd ed.). Thousand Oaks, CA: SAGE.

Cooper, H., Hedges, L. V., & Valentine, J. C. (Eds.). (2009). *The handbook of research synthesis and meta-analysis* (2nd ed.). New York: Russell Sage Foundation.

Council of Writing Program Administrators. (2003). Defining and avoiding plagiarism: The WPA statement on best practices. Retrieved from *http://wpacouncil.org/positions/WPAplagiarism.pdf*.

Creswell, J. W. (2012). *Qualitative inquiry and research design: Choosing among five traditions* (3rd ed.). Thousand Oaks, CA: SAGE.

Creswell, J. W. (2018). *Research design: Qualitative, quantitative, and mixed methods approaches* (5th ed.). Thousand Oaks, CA: SAGE.

Creswell, J. W., & Plano Clark, V. L. (2011). *Designing and conducting mixed methods research* (2nd ed.). Thousand Oaks, CA: SAGE.

Daley, B. J., & Torre, D. M. (2010). Concept maps in medical education: An analytical literature review. *Medical Education, 44*(5), 440–448.

Daly, J. A., & Miller, M. D. (1975). Apprehension of writing as a predictor of message intensity. *Journal of Psychology, 89*(2), 175–177.

Danica, S., Ventura, A., & Verdaguer, I. (2013). A cross-disciplinary analysis of personal and impersonal features in English and Spanish scientific writing. In I. Verdaguer, N. J. Laso, & S. Danica (Eds.), *Biomedical English: A corpus-based approach* (pp. 121–143). Philadelphia: John Benjamin.

Dawidowicz, P. (2010). *Literature review made easy: A quick guide to success.* Charlotte, NC: Information Age.

DeGue, S., Valle, L. A., Holt, M. K., Massetti, G. M., Jatjasko, J. L., & Tharp, A. T. (2014). A systematic review of primary prevention strategies for sexual violence perpetration. *Aggression and Violent Behavior, 19*, 346–362.

Denzin, N. K. (2009). The elephant in the living room: Or extending the conversation about the politics of evidence. *Qualitative Research, 9*(2), 139–160.

Denzin, N. K., & Lincoln, Y. S. (Eds.). (2011). *The SAGE handbook of qualitative research* (4th ed.). Thousand Oaks, CA: SAGE.

Dewar, M. D. (2015). *Uncovering being from the well: Recovering meaning in education through a phenomenology of well-being.* Unpublished doctoral dissertation, National Louis University, Chicago, IL.

Dixon-Woods, M., Bonas, S., Booth, A., Jones, D. R., Miller, T., Sutton, A. J., et al. (2006). How can systematic reviews incorporate qualitative research?: A critical perspective. *Qualitative Research, 6*(1), 27–44.

Dixon-Woods, M., Cavers, D., Agarwal, S., Annandale, E., Arthur, A., Harvey, J., et al. (2006). Conducting a critical interpretive review of the literature on access to healthcare by vulnerable groups. *BMC Medical Research Methodology, 6*, 35.

Dixon-Woods, M., Shaw, R. L., Agarwal, S., & Smith, J. A. (2004). The problem of appraising qualitative research. *Quality and Safety in Healthcare, 13*, 223–225.

Dong, Y. R. (1998). Nonnative graduate students' thesis dissertation writing in science: Self reports of students and their advisors from two US institutes. *English for Specific Purposes, 17*(4), 369–390.

Douglas, J. (2014). Making a case in your literature review. In A. J. Rockinson-Szapkiw & L.

S. Spaulding (Eds.), *Navigating the doctoral journey: A handbook of strategies for success* (pp. 139–148). Lanham, MD: Rowman & Littlefield.

Doyle, L. H. (2003). Synthesis through meta-ethnography: Paradoxes, enhancements and possibilities. *Qualitative Research, 3*(3), 321–344.

Driscoll, D. L., & Brizee, A. (2015). Quoting, paraphrasing, and summarizing (Purdue Online Writing Lab). Retrieved from *https://owl.english.purdue.edu/owl/resource/563/1.*

Dweck, C. S. (2016, January 13). What having a "growth mindset" actually means. *Harvard Business Review.* Retrieved from *https://hbr.org/2016/01/what-having-a-growth-mindset-actually-means.*

Dykiert, D. (2014). *Data extraction, quality assessment and narrative synthesis.* Edinburgh, UK: Centre for Cognitive Ageing and Cognitive Epidemiology, University of Edinburgh. Retrieved from *www.ccace.ed.ac.uk/sites/default/files/Data%20extraction,%20assessment%20and%20synthesis_2014.pdf.*

Efron, S. E. (2015, April). *Moral dialogue with self and with others.* Paper presented at the annual meeting of the American Educational Research Association, Chicago, IL.

Efron, S. E., & Ravid, R. (2013). *Action research in education: A practical guide.* New York: Guilford Press.

Efron, S. E., Winter, J., & Bressman, S. (2017). Mentoring across cultures: Supporting relationships that inspire professional growth. In A. M. Kent & A. M. Green (Eds.), *Across the domains: Examining best practices in mentoring public school education* (pp. 69–96). Charlotte, NC: Information Age.

Elbow, P. (1973). *Writing without teachers.* New York: Oxford University Press.

Elbow, P. (1998). *Writing with power: Techniques for mastering the writing process* (2nd ed.). New York: Oxford University Press.

Elbow, P. (2000). *Everyone can write: Essays toward a hopeful theory of writing and teaching writing.* New York: Oxford University Press.

Elbow, P., & Belanoff, P. (1995). *A community of writers: A workshop course in writing* (2nd ed.). New York: McGraw-Hill.

Feak, C. B., & Swales, J. M. (2009). *Telling a research story: Writing a literature review.* Ann Arbor: University of Michigan Press.

Fisher, A. (2004). *The logic of real arguments* (2nd ed.). Cambridge, UK: Cambridge University Press.

Flick, W. (2009). *An introduction to qualitative research* (4th ed.). Thousand Oaks, CA: SAGE.

Forte, J. (2010). Transformation through interaction: A meta-ethnographic synthesis of research reports on mutual aid groups. *Qualitative Social Work, 9*(2), 151–168.

Francel, J. (2015). *The war on education: A prisoner's dilemma.* Unpublished doctoral dissertation, National Louis University, Chicago, IL.

Gadamer, H. G. (1982). *Truth and method* (G. Barden & J. Cumming, Trans.). New York: Crossroads.

Gadamer, H. G. (1998). *Truth and method* (2nd ed.) (J. Weinsheimer & D. Marshall, Trans.). New York: Continuum. (Original work published 1960)

Gadamer, H. G. (2004). *Truth and method.* New York: Continuum International.

Gall, M. D., Gall, J. P., & Borg, W. R. (2006). *Educational research: An introduction* (8th ed.). Upper Saddle River, NJ: Pearson.

Galvan, J. L., & Galvan, M. C. (2017). *Writing literature reviews: A guide for students of the social and behavioral sciences* (6th ed.). New York: Routledge.

Ganann, R., Ciliska, D., & Thomas, H. (2010). Expediting systematic reviews: Methods and implications of rapid reviews. *Implementation Science, 5*, 56.

Garrard, J. (2014). *Health sciences literature review made easy: The matrix method* (4th ed.). Burlington, MA: Jones & Bartlett Learning.

Gay, L. R., Mills, G. E., & Airasian, P. W. (2011). *Educational research: Competencies for analysis and applications* (10th ed.). Boston: Addison-Wesley.

Geertz, C. (1979). From the native's point of view: The nature of anthropological understanding. In P. Rabinow & W. M. Sullivan (Eds.), *Interpretive social science: A reader* (pp. 225–241). Berkeley: University of California Press.

Glass, G. (1976). Primary, secondary, and meta-analysis of research. *Educational Researcher, 5*(10), 3–8.

Glense, C. (2018). *Becoming qualitative researchers: An introduction* (4th ed.). New York: Pearson.

Goldhaber, D., Lavery, L., & Theobald, R. (2015). Uneven playing field?: Assessing the teacher quality gap between advantaged and disadvantaged students. *Educational Researcher, 44*(5), 293–307.

Goodson, P. (2013). *Becoming an academic writer: 50 exercises for paced, productive, and powerful writing.* Thousand Oaks, CA: SAGE.

Gough, D. (2007). Weight of evidence: A framework for the appraisal of the quality and relevance of evidence. In J. Furlong & A. Oancea (Eds.), Applied and practice-based research [Special issue]. *Research Papers in Education, 22*(2), 213–228.

Gough, D., Oliver, S., & Thomas, J. (Eds.). (2012). *An introduction to systematic reviews.* Thousand Oaks, CA: SAGE.

Graff, G., & Birkenstein, C. (2014). *They say/I say: The moves that matter in academic writing* (3rd ed.). New York: Norton.

Grant, J., Ling, T., Potoglou, D., & Culley, D. M. (2011). A report prepared by RAND Europe for the Greek Ministry of Education, Lifelong learning and religious affairs. Retrieved from *www.rand.org/content/dam/rand/pubs/documented_briefings/2011/RAND_DB631.pdf.*

Greene, M. (1978). *Landscapes of learning.* New York: Teachers College Press.

Gunn, K. C. M., & Delafield-Butt, J. T. (2016). Teaching children with autism spectrum disorder with restricted interests: A review of evidence for best practice. *Review of Educational Research, 86*(2), 408–430.

Hammersley, M. (2000). Varieties of social research. *International Journal of Social Research Methodology: Theory and Practice, 3*(3), 221–231.

Hammersley, M. (2007). The issue of quality in qualitative research. *International Journal of Research and Method in Education, 30*(2), 27–44.

Han, Y. C., & Love, J. (2015). Stages of immigrant parent involvement—survivors to leaders. *Phi Delta Kappan, 97*(4), 21–25.

Hannes, K. (2011). Critical appraisal of qualitative research. In J. Noyes, A. Booth, K. Hannes, A. Harden, J. Harris, S. Lewin, et al. (Eds.), *Supplementary guidance for inclusion of qualitative research in Cochrane Systematic Reviews of Interventions* (Version 1, updated August 2011). Cochrane Collaboration Qualitative Methods Group. Retrieved from *http://cqrmg.cochrane.org/supplemental-handbook-guidance.*

Hannes, K. (2015). Building a case for mixed method review. In D. Richards & I. Hallberg (Eds.), *Complex interventions in health: An overview of research methods* (pp. 88–95). Oxon, UK: Routledge.

Harden, A., & Thomas, J. (2005). Methodological issues in combining diverse study types in systematic reviews. *International Journal of Social Research Methodology, 8*(3), 257–271.

Harden, A., & Thomas, J. (2010). Mixed methods and systematic reviews: Examples and emerging issues. In A. Tashakkori & C. Teddlie (Eds.), *Handbook of mixed methods in the social and behavioral sciences* (2nd ed., pp. 749–774). London: SAGE.

Harker J., & Kleijnen, J. (2012). What is rapid review?: A methodological exploration of rapid reviews in health technology assessments. *International Journal of Evidence-Based Health Care, 10*(4), 397–410.

Hart, C. (1998). *Doing the literature search: Releasing the social science research imagination.* London: SAGE.

Hart, C. (2001). *Doing a literature search: A comprehensive guide for the social sciences* (W. McNeil & N. Walker, Trans.). Los Angeles: SAGE.

Heidegger, M. (1995). *The fundamental concept of metaphysics: World, finitude, and solitude.* Bloomington: Indiana University Press.

Hesse-Biber, S. N. (2010). *Mixed methods research: Merging theory with practice.* New York: Guilford Press.

Heyvaert, M., Maes, B., & Onghena, P. (2013). Mixed methods research synthesis: Definition, framework, and potential. *Quality and Quantity, 47*, 659–676.

Higgins, J., & Green, S. (Eds.). (2011). *Cochrane handbook for systematic reviews of interventions.* Chichester, UK: Wiley.

Holstein, J. A., & Gubrium, J. F. (Eds.). (2012). *Varieties of narrative analysis.* Thousand Oaks, CA: SAGE.

Issel, L. M. (2014). *Health program planning and evaluation: A practical, systematic approach for community health* (3rd ed.). Burlington, MA: Jones & Bartlett Learning.

Jarret, M. A., & Ollendick, T. H. (2008). A conceptual review of the comorbidity of attention-deficit/hyperactivity disorder and anxiety: Implications for future research and practice. *Clinical Psychology Review, 28*, 1266–1280.

Jesson, J., Matheson, L., & Lacey, F. M. (2011). *Doing your literature review: Traditional and systematic techniques.* Thousand Oaks, CA: SAGE.

Johnson, B., & Christensen, L. (2010). *Educational research: Quantitative, qualitative, and mixed approaches* (4th ed.). Thousand Oaks, CA: SAGE.

Johnson, B. R., & Onwuegbuzie, A. J. (2004). Mixed methods research: A research paradigm whose time has come. *Educational Researcher, 33*(7), 14–26.

Jordan, A. D. (2015). *The transformative experiences of female educators as a catalyst for social change in the world.* Unpublished doctoral dissertation, National Louis University, Chicago, IL.

Kafle, N. P. (2011). Hermeneutic phenomenological research method simplified. *BODHI International Journal of Research in Humanities, Arts and Science, 5*(1), 181–200.

Kalmer, B., & Thomson, P. (2006). *Helping doctoral students write: Pedagogies for doctoral supervision.* London: Routledge.

Kalmer, B., & Thomson, P. (2008). *The failure of dissertation advice books: Toward alternative pedagogies for doctoral supervision.* London: Routledge.

Kent, A. M., Kochan, F., & Green, A. M. (2013). Cultural influences on mentoring programs and relationships. A critical review of research. *International Journal of Mentoring and Coaching in Education, 2*(3), 204–217.

Koricheva, J., & Gurevitch, J. (2013). Place of meta-analysis among other methods of research synthesis. In J. Koricheva, J. Gurevitch, & K. Mengersen (Eds.), *Handbook of meta-analysis in ecology and evolution* (pp. 3–13). Princeton, NJ: Princeton University Press.

Kwan, B. S. C. (2008). The nexus of reading, writing, and researching in the doctoral undertaking of humanities and social sciences: Implications for literature reviewing. *English for Specific Purposes, 27*(1), 42–56.

Langdridge, D. (2007). *Phenomenological psychology: Theory, research and method.* New York: Pearson.

Lau, J., Ioannidis, J. P. A., & Schmid, C. H. (1997). Quantitative synthesis in systematic reviews. *American College of Physicians, 127*(9), 820–826.

Laverty, S. M. (2003). Hermeneutic phenomenology and phenomenology: A comparison of historical and methodological considerations. *International Journal of Qualitative Methods, 2*(3), Article 3.

Lazonder, A. W., & Harmsen, R. (2016). Meta-analysis of inquiry-based learning. *Review of Educational Research, 86*(3), 681–718.

Lee, R. P., Hart, R. I., Watson, R. M., & Rapley, T. (2015). Qualitative synthesis in practice: Some pragmatics of meta-ethnography. *Qualitative Research, 15*(3), 334–350.

Lichtman, M. V. (2013). *Qualitative research for the social science.* Thousand Oaks, CA: SAGE.

Lincoln, Y. S., & Guba, E. G. (1985). *Naturalistic inquiry.* Newbury Park, CA: SAGE.

Lockwood, C., & Pearson, A. (2013). *A comparison of meta-aggregation and meta-ethnography as qualitative review methods.* Adelaide, Australia: Joanna Briggs Institute.

Lomask, M. (1987). *The biographer's craft.* New York: Harper and Row.

Lukenchuk, A. (Ed.). (2013). *Paradigms of research for the 21st century: Perspectives and examples from practice.* New York: Peter Lang.

Lynch, T. (2014). *Writing up your PhD (qualitative research): Independent study version.* Edinburgh, UK: English Language Teacher Center, University of Edinburgh.

Machi, L. A., & McEvoy, B. T. (2012). *The literature review: Six steps to success* (2nd ed.). New York: Corwin.

Magrini, J. M. (2014). *Being-in-the-world as being-with-others-in-learning: How the analytic of original learning unfolds as a hermeneutic of existence.* Unpublished doctoral dissertation, National Louis University, Chicago, IL.

Makambi, K. (2012). *Alternative methods for meta-analysis.* Saarbrucken, Germany: LAP Lambert Academic.

Marshall, C., & Rossman, G. B. (2015). *Designing qualitative research* (6th ed.). Thousand Oaks, CA: SAGE.

Maxwell, J. A. (2006). Literature reviews of, and for, educational research: A commentary on Boote and Beile's "Scholars before researchers." *Educational Researcher, 35*(9), 28–31.

Maxwell, J. A. (2013). *Qualitative research design: An interactive approach* (3rd ed.). Thousand Oaks, CA: SAGE.

Mays, T. L., & Smith, B. (2009). Navigating the doctoral journey. *Journal of Hospital Library Scholarship, 9,* 345–361.

McDonald, J. H. (2014). *Handbook of biological statistics* (3rd ed.). Baltimore: Sparky House.

McMillan, J. H., & Schumacher, S. (2010). *Research in education: Evidence-based inquiry* (7th ed.). Boston: Pearson.

McMillan, J. H., & Wergin, J. F. (2010). *Understanding and evaluating educational research* (4th ed.). Boston: Pearson.

Menager-Beeley, R., & Paulos, L. (2006). *Understanding plagiarism: A student guide to writing your own work*. Boston: Houghton Mifflin.

Merriam, S. B. (2009). *Qualitative research: A guide to designing and implementation*. San Francisco: Jossey-Bass.

Merriam, S. B., & Tisdell, E. J. (2016). *Qualitative research: A guide to designing and implementation* (4th ed.). San Francisco: Jossey-Bass.

Mertler, C. A. (2012). *Action research: Improving schools and empowering educators* (3rd ed.). Los Angeles: SAGE.

Miles, M. B., Huberman, A. M., & Saldaña, J. (2013). *Qualitative data analysis: A methods sourcebook* (3rd ed.). Thousand Oaks, CA: SAGE.

Miller, T., & Birch, M. (Eds.). (2012). *Ethics in qualitative research*. Thousand Oaks, CA: SAGE.

Modern Language Association. (2016). *MLA handbook for writers of research papers* (7th ed.). New York: Author.

Myers, M. D. (2004). Hermeneutics in information systems research. In J. Minges & L. P. Wilcock (Eds.), *Social theory and philosophy for information systems* (pp. 103–128). Chichester, UK: Wiley.

Noblit, G. W., & Hare, R. D. (1988). *Meta-ethnography: Synthesizing qualitative studies*. Newbury Park, CA: SAGE.

Nolte, M. C., Bruce, M. A., & Becker, K. W. (2014). Building a community of researchers using research mentoring model. *Journal of Counselor Preparation and Supervision, 7*(2), Article 1.

Ollhoff, J. (2013). *How to write a literature review: Workbook in six steps*. Farmington, MN: Sparrow Media Group.

Onwuegbuzie, A. J., & Frels, R. (2016). *Seven steps to a comprehensive literature review: A multimodal and cultural approach*. Thousand Oaks, CA: SAGE.

Paiz, J. M., Angeli, E., Wagner, J., Lawrick, E., Moore, K., Anderson, M., et al. (2016, May 13). General format. Purdue Online Writing Lab. Retrieved from *https://owl.english.purdue.edu/owl/resource/560/02*.

Pallini, S., Baiocco, R., Schneider, B. H., Madigan, S., & Atkinson, L. (2014). Early child–parent attachment and peer relations: A meta-analysis of recent research. *Journal of Family Psychology, 28*(1), 118–123.

Pan, M. L. (2013). *Preparing literature reviews: Qualitative and quantitative approaches* (4th ed.). Los Angeles: Pyrczak.

Park, C. L. (2010). Making sense of meaning literature: An integrative review of meaning making and its effects on adjustment to stressful life events. *Psychological Bulletin, 136*(2), 257–301.

Patterson, M. E., & Williams, D. R. (2002). *Advances in tourism applications series: Vol. 9. Collecting and analyzing qualitative data: Hermeneutic principles, methods and case examples*. Champaign, IL: Sagamore.

Petticrew, M., & Roberts, H. (2005). *Systematic reviews in social sciences: A practical guide*. Malden, MA: Blackwell.

Platridge, B. (2002). Thesis and dissertation writing: An examination of published advice and actual practice. *English for Specific Purposes, 21*, 125–143.

Pluye, P., & Hong, Q. N. (2014). Combining the power of stories and the power of numbers: Mixed methods review and mixed studies review. *Annual Review of Public Health, 35*, 29–45.

Polit, D. F., & Beck, C. T. (2013). *Essential of nursing research: Appraising evidence for nursing practice.* Philadelphia: Wolters Kluwer/Lippincott Williams & Wilkins.

Polkinghorne, D. (1983). *Methodology for human science: Systems of inquiry.* Albany: State University of New York Press.

Pope, C., Mays, N., & Popay, J. (2007). *Synthesizing qualitative and quantitative health evidence: A guide to methods.* New York: Open University Press.

Quinn, D. M., & Cooc, N. (2015). Science achievement gaps by gender and race/ethnicity in elementary and middle school: Trends and predictors. *Educational Researcher, 44*(6), 336–346.

Ramanigopal, C. S., Palaniappan, C., & Mani, A. (2012). Mind mapping and knowledge management: Coding and implementation of knowledge. *International Journal of Management, 3*(2), 250–259.

Randolph, J. (2009). A guide to writing the dissertation literature review. *Practical Assessment, Research and Evaluation, 14*(13), 1–13.

Ravid, L. (2015). *Medical innovation in the Civil War era.* Unpublished manuscript.

Ravid, R. (2015). *Practical statistics for educators* (5th ed.). Lanham, MD: Rowman & Littlefield.

Ravitch, S. M., & Riggan, M. (2017). *Reason and rigor: How conceptual frameworks guide research* (2nd ed.). Thousand Oaks, CA: SAGE.

Reid, H. M. (2014). *Introduction to statistics: Fundamental concepts and procedures of data analysis.* Los Angeles: SAGE.

Reiff, P. (2016). *Refreshment for the soul: A phenomenological study of the student experience of beauty in school.* Unpublished doctoral dissertation, National Louis University, Chicago, IL.

Richards, L. (2009). *Handling qualitative data: A practical guide* (2nd ed.). Thousand Oaks, CA: SAGE.

Richardson, L. (1990). *Writing strategies: Reaching diverse audiences (qualitative research methods).* Newbury Park, CA: SAGE.

Richardson, L., & St. Pierre, E. A. (2005). Writing: A method of inquiry. In N. K. Denzin & Y. S. Lincoln (Eds.), *The Sage handbook of qualitative research* (3rd ed., pp. 923–948). Thousand Oaks, CA: SAGE.

Ricoeur, P. (1981). *The rule of metaphor: Multi-disciplinary studies of the creation of meaning in language* (R. Czerny, Trans.). Toronto: University of Toronto Press.

Ridley, D. (2012). *The literature review: A step by step guide for students* (2nd ed.). Thousand Oaks, CA: SAGE.

Ringquist, E. (2013). *Meta-analysis for public management and policy.* Hoboken, NJ: Wiley.

Rocco, T. S., & Plakhotnik, M. S. (2009). Literature reviews, conceptual frameworks, and theoretical frameworks: Terms, functions, and distinctions. *Human Resource Development Review, 8*(1), 120.

Romano, T. (2004). *Crafting authentic voice.* Portsmouth, NH: Heinemann.

Rosenthal, R. (1979). The "file drawer problem" and tolerance for null results. *Psychological Bulletin, 86*(3), 638–641.

Rothstein, H. R., Sutton, A. J., & Borenstein, M. (Eds.). (2005). *Publication bias in meta-analysis: Prevention, assessment and adjustments.* Hoboken, NJ: Wiley.

Saini, M., & Shlonsky, A. (2012). *Systematic synthesis of qualitative research.* New York: Oxford University Press.

Sandelowski, M., Voils, C. I., & Barroso, J. (2006). Defining and designing mixed research synthesis studies. *Research in the Schools, 13,* 29–40.

Sarasin, K. (2017). *A suburban case of community mobilization for music education: Lessons for art education in a cash-strapped world.* Unpublished manuscript.

Schick-Makaroff, K., MacDonald, M., Plummer, M., Burgess, J., & Neander, W. (2016). What synthesis methodology should I use?: A review and analysis of approaches to research synthesis. *AIMS Public Health, 3*(1), 172–215.

Schmidt, F. L., & Hunter, J. E. (2015). *Methods of meta-analysis: Correcting error and bias in research findings* (3rd ed.). Thousand Oaks, CA: SAGE.

Schulman, L. S. (1999). Professing educational scholarship. In E. C. Lagemann & L. S. Schulman (Eds.), *Issues in education research: Problems and possibilities* (pp. 159–165). San Francisco: Jossey-Bass.

Schutz, A. (1967). *Phenomenology of the social world* (G. Walsh & F. Lehnert, Trans.). Evanston, IL: Northwestern University Press.

Shaw, C. (2010). Writer's voice: The gateway to dialogue. *SFU Educational Review, 4,* 4–12.

Sherman, B. S. (2014). *Scholarship students: Squeezing through the glass ceiling of an affluent private school.* Unpublished doctoral dissertation, National Louis University, Chicago, IL.

Silverman, D. (2015). *Interpreting qualitative data* (5th ed.). Thousand Oaks, CA: SAGE.

Slattery, P. (2013). *Curriculum development in the postmodern era: Teaching and learning in an age of accountability* (3rd ed.). New York: Routledge.

Slavin, R. E. (2007). *Educational research in an age of accountability.* Boston: Pearson.

Smith, D. G. (1991). Hermeneutic inquiry: The hermeneutic imagination and the pedagogic text. In E. C. Short (Ed.), *Forms of curriculum inquiry* (pp. 187–210). Albany: State University of New York Press.

Smythe, E., & Spence, D. (2012). Re-viewing literature in hermeneutic research. *International Journal of Qualitative Methods, 11*(1), 12–25.

Song, F., Parekh-Bhurke, S., Hooper, L., Loke, Y. K., Ryder, J. J., Sutton, A. J., et al. (2009). Extent of publication bias in different categories of research cohorts: A meta-analysis of empirical studies. *BMC Medical Research Methodology, 9,* 79.

Strike, K., & Posner, G. (1983). Types of synthesis and their criteria. In S. A. Ward & L. J. Reed (Eds.), *Knowledge structure and use* (pp. 343–362). Philadelphia: Temple University Press.

Sullivan, A. L., & Simonson, G. R. (2016). A systematic review of school-based social-emotional interventions for refugee and war-traumatized youth. *Review of Educational Research, 86*(2), 503–530.

Suri, H. (2011). Purposeful sampling in qualitative research synthesis. *Qualitative Research Journal, 11*(2), 63–75.

Tan, E. (2014). Human capital theory: A holistic criticism. *Review of Educational Research, 84*(3), 411–445.

Tashakkori, A., & Teddlie, C. B. (Eds.). (2010). *SAGE handbook of mixed methods in social and behavioral sciences.* Thousand Oaks, CA: SAGE.

Taylor, C. N., & Kilgus, S. P. (2014). Social–emotional learning. *Principal Leadership, 15*(1), 12–16.

Teddlie, C. B., & Tashakkori, A. M. (2009). *Foundations of mixed methods research: Integrating quantitative and qualitative approaches in the social and behavioral sciences.* Thousand Oaks, CA: SAGE.

Tessema, M. T., Ready, K. J., & Astani, M. (2014). Does a part-time job affect college students' satisfaction and academic performance (GPA)? The case of a mid-sized public university. *International Journal of Business Administration, 5*(2), 50–59.

Thompson, P. (1999). Exploring the contexts of writing: Interview with PhD supervisors. In P. Thompson (Ed.), *Issues in EAP writing research and instruction* (pp. 37–54). Reading, UK: University of Reading Center of Applied Language Studies.

Torraco, R. J. (2005). Writing integrative literature review: Guidelines and examples. *Human Resource Development Review, 4,* 356–367.

Toulmin, S. E. (2003). *The uses of argument.* Cambridge, UK: Cambridge University Press.

Toye, F., Seers, K., Alcoke, N., Briggs, M., Carr, E., & Barker, K (2014). Meta-ethnography 25 years on: Challenges and insights for synthesizing a large number of qualitative studies. *BMC Medical Research Methodology, 14,* 80.

Uman, L. S. (2011). Systematic reviews and meta-analyses. *Journal of the Canadian Academy of Child and Adolescent Psychiatry, 20*(1), 57–59.

van Manen, M. (1990). *Researching lived experience: Human science for an action sensitive pedagogy* (2nd ed.). Albany: State University of New York Press.

van Manen, M. (2014). *Phenomenology of practice: Meaning-giving methods in phenomenological research and writing.* Walnut Creek, CA: Left Coast Press.

Vanhoozer, K. J., Smith, J. K. A., & Bonson, B. E. (2006). *Hermeneutics at a crossroad.* Bloomington: Indiana University Press.

Viechtbauer, W., & Cheung M. (2010). Outlier and influence diagnostics for meta-analysis. *Research Synthesis Methods, 1,* 112–125.

Walsh, D., & Downe, S. (2005). Meta-synthesis method for qualitative research: A literature review. *Journal of Advanced Nursing, 50*(2), 204–211.

Walton, D. N. (2013). *Methods of argumentation.* New York: Cambridge University Press.

Wellington, J., Bathmaker, A., Hunt, C., McCulloch, G., & Sikes, P. (2005). *Succeeding with your doctorate.* London: SAGE.

What Is Citation? (n.d.). Retrieved January 5, 2016, from *http://plagiarism.org/citing-sources/whats-a-citation.*

Whittemore, R., & Knafl, K. (2005). The integrative review: Updated methodology. *Journal of Advanced Nursing, 52*(5), 546–553.

Wieman, C. E. (2007). Why not try a scientific approach to science education? *Change, 39*(5), 9–15.

Wieman, C. E. (2014). The similarities between research in education and research in the hard sciences. *Educational Researcher, 43*(1), 12–14.

Winkler-Wagner, R. (2015). Having their lives narrowed down?: The state of black women's college success. *Review of Educational Research, 85*(2), 171–204.

Wisker, G. (2015). Developing doctoral authors: Engaging with theoretical perspectives through the literature review. *Innovations in Education and Teaching International, 52*(1), 64–74.

Wisker, G., & Savin-Baden, M. (2009). Priceless conceptual threshold: Beyond the "stuck place" in writing. *London Review of Education, 7*(3), 235–247.

Wolcott, E. H. (2009). *Writing up qualitative research* (3rd ed.). Thousand Oaks, CA: SAGE.

Yin, R. K. (2015). *Qualitative research from start to finish* (2nd ed.). New York: Guilford Press.

Yoon, E., Chang, C., Kim, S., Clawson, A., Cleary, S. E., Hansen, M., et al. (2013). A meta-analysis of acculturation/enculturation and mental health. *Journal of Counseling Psychology, 60*(1), 15–30.

Yu, C. H. (2006). *Philosophical foundations of quantitative research methodology.* Lanham, MD: University Press of America.

SOFTWARE PROGRAMS AND WEBSITES

Software Programs

COMPAS: *www.softschools.com/teacher_resources/concept_map_maker*

FreeMind: *www.freemind.sourceforge.net*

Inspirato: *www.inspiration.com*

Lucidchart: *www.lucidchart.com/pages*

MindGenius: *www.mindgenius.com/default.aspx*

Mindmeister: *www.mindmeister.com*

MindMup: *www.mindmup.com/#m:offline-map-1*

MindView: *www.matchware.com/en/products/mindview/mindviewonline.htm*

SmartDraw: *www.smartdraw.com*

Websites

Amazon: *www.amazon.com*

EBSCO system: *www.ebscohost.com*

Elsevier (which includes Scopus): *www.elsevier.com/solutions/scopus*

EndNote: *http://endnote.com*

ERIC: *http://eric.ed.gov*

Goodreads: *www.goodreads.com/author/quotes/1498146.Linton_Weeks*

Google Scholar: *http://scholar.google.com*

ProQuest: *www.proquest.com*

PsycINFO: *www.apa.org/pubs/databases/psycinfo/index.aspx*

Purdue University Owl website: *https://owl.english.purdue.edu/owl*

Style Wizard: *www.stylewizard.com*

Turnitin: *http://turnitin.com*

U.S. Department of Education: *www.ed.gov*

Zotero: *www.zotero.org/about*

Index

Note. *f*, *t*, or *b* following a page number indicates a figure, table, or box.

About the Authors

Sara Efrat Efron, EdD, is Professor of Education and Director of the Doctoral Program in Curriculum, Advocacy and Policy at National Louis University. Her areas of interest include teacher research, mentoring, and moral and democratic education in times of crisis. Dr. Efron is coauthor with Ruth Ravid of *Action Research in Education*. She has published numerous book chapters and journal articles and presents widely at national and international conferences. She has also written several foreign-language instruction books for middle and high school students.

Ruth Ravid, PhD, is Professor Emerita of Education at National Louis University. Her areas of interest include educational research, action research, assessment, and school–university collaboration. Dr. Ravid has authored and edited eight books, including a practical guide coauthored with Sara Efrat Efron, *Action Research in Education*, as well as numerous journal articles and book chapters.